ORTHOPAEDIA:

SPORTS MEDICINE

Produced by:

THE CODMAN GROUP

A 503C Non-profit committed to enhancing medical education, patient care, and research through the promotion of collaboration, the open exchange of data and content, and the transmission of knowledge across academic networks.

CONTENTS

SERIES INTRODUCTION

Orthopaedia is produced by The Codman Group (a 503C IRS-approved public charity) in collaboration with the United States Bone and Joint Initiative and the Community of Musculoskeletal Educators. ***Orthopaedia*** aims to serve as a free, up-to-date, peer-reviewed open educational resource for students and practitioners, thereby improving the welfare of patients.

Please visit *http://www.orthopaedia.com* for the most current version of this text. At the website, you will also find its sister publications covering Hand and Foot & Ankle disorders, and others as they become available.

Dan Jacob
President, The Codman Group

Joseph Bernstein, MD, FACS
Stephen J. Pinney, MD, MEd, FRCS(C)
Christian Veillette, MD, FRCS(C)
Orthopaedia Series Editors

PREFACE

The study of sports medicine is perhaps the most interesting of the orthopaedic specialties. Within this field is the tremendous hope of mankind: namely, to change the course of natural history. With every passing day, we lose chondrocytes, osteocytes, and tenocytes to the ravages of wear and tear. Unlocking the mystery of cartilage, bone, and soft tissue regeneration is the next frontier of orthopaedic science, and one in which the sports medicine physician is thoroughly engaged. Through our evolving understanding of the biologic processes of the musculoskeletal system, the sports medicine physician is constantly adherent to the adage, 'function follows form.' It is the field of sports medicine that took the moon shot in orthopaedics, namely, to re-create damaged anatomy to its native state.

From the medical student perspective, the field of sports medicine is really where one should begin. While it is certainly intriguing to think of sports medicine as a specialty whose sole concern is getting athletes back to their craft, it is really much more. The sports medicine physician is the true diagnostician of the musculoskeletal world. If you had a musculoskeletal problem, but weren't sure where to go first, I'd say you should start with a sports medicine specialist.

As you explore this volume covering the most common conditions that sports specialists treat, I hope you will see exactly what I mean. There is no part of the musculoskeletal system that isn't known to the sports medicine surgeon. Whether it is the spine, foot and ankle, or shoulder, we've got it covered.

This volume is our best attempt to make the information digestible, practical, easy to understand, and current. It should be where every medical student begins his or her journey in orthopaedics. There is no question that there will be chapters here that will, sooner or later apply to you or someone you know. It is for this reason that sports medicine is so relevant, and key to any foundational knowledge in musculoskeletal disease.

Fotios Paul Tjoumakaris, MD
Associate Professor, Orthopaedic Surgery
Sidney Kimmel College of Medicine, Thomas Jefferson University
Rothman Orthopaedic Institute
Associate Director, Sports Medicine Fellowship, Thomas Jefferson University
Philadelphia, PA

A WORD ON PEER REVIEW

There is a great profusion of medical information available for free on the Internet, and a lot of it is good. Yet even good information may not be completely useful to the reader who may not know if it is trustworthy. By contrast, there is also a lot of medical information available for sale that is produced by well-known authors and organizations, though not always for free. This volume aims to be both free and authoritative.

To ensure medical accuracy, all of the material was reviewed by the section editors, who are of course content experts of great renown. In addition, each chapter was reviewed by an expert who was not involved in the creation of the material. These reviewers were asked to read the chapter with one overriding goal in mind: to detect errors. The reviewers were then asked to "certify" the chapter as a reasonable presentation of the topic without any glaring mistakes in content. We are grateful to our reviewers, listed below:

- Christopher Arena, MD reviewed Achilles Tendon Disorders. Dr. Arena is an Orthopaedic Surgeon affiliated with the Penn State Bone & Joint Institute.
- Nicole Belkin, MD reviewed Disorders of the Collateral Ligaments and Cruciate Ligament Injuries of the Knee. Dr. Belkin is an orthopaedic surgeon and sports medicine specialist at Columbia University.
- James Carey, MD reviewed Meniscus Tears and Chondral Injuries of the Knee. Dr. Carey is an orthopaedic surgeon and sports medicine specialist at the University of Pennsylvania.
- Michael Castro, DO reviewed Ankle Sprains. Dr. Castro is a Foot and Ankle Orthopaedic Surgeon at Summit Orthopedics.
- Steven Cohen, MD reviewed Disorders of the Elbow Ligaments and Osteochondral Injuries of the Elbow. Dr. Cohen is an orthopaedic surgeon and sports medicine specialist at the Rothman Institute.
- Kevin Freedman, MD reviewed Patellofemoral Pain and Patellar Instability. Dr. Freedman is an orthopaedic surgeon and sports medicine specialist at the Rothman Institute.
- Sommer Hammoud, MD reviewed Adhesive Capsulitis and Glenohumeral Instability. Dr. Hammoud is an orthopaedic surgeon and sports medicine specialist at the Rothman Institute.
- Paul Juliano, MD reviewed Achilles Tendon Disorders. Dr Juliano is a Foot and Ankle Orthopaedic Surgeon, Professor, Vice Chairman, Residency Director at Penn States Hershey Bone and Joint Institute.
- Rahul Kapur, MD reviewed Stress Fractures and the Female Athletic Triad. Dr Kapur is a family and sports medicine physician at the University of Minnesota.
- John D. Kelly IV, MD reviewed Scapulothoracic Disorders. Dr. Kelly is an orthopaedic surgeon and sports medicine specialist at the University of Pennsylvania.
- Andrew Kuntz, MD reviewed Epicondylitis of the Elbow. Dr. Kuntz is a fellowship trained shoulder and elbow surgeon at the University of PA.
- Andrew Milby, MD reviewed Burners and Stingers and Spondylolysis and Spondylolisthesis. Dr. Milby is a spine surgeon at Emory University.
- Kevin O'Donnell, MD reviewed Disorders of the Rotator Cuff and Glenohumeral Arthritis. Dr. O'Donnell is an orthopaedic surgeon and sports medicine specialist in private practice.
- John Salvo, MD reviewed Tendon Disorders of the Hip and Thigh and Labral Tears of the Hip and Femoroacetabular Impingement. Dr. Salvo is an orthopaedic surgeon and sports medicine specialist at the Rothman Institute.

- John Scolaro, MD reviewed Proximal Humerus Fractures and Clavicle Fractures. Dr. Scolaro is an orthopaedic traumatologist at the University of California, Irvine.
- Fotios Tjoumakaris, MD reviewed Disorders of the Biceps and Triceps. Dr. Tjoumakaris is an orthopaedic surgeon and sports medicine specialist at the Rothman Institute.
- Bradford Tucker, MD reviewed Disorders of the Extensor Mechanism. Dr. Tucker is an orthopaedic surgeon and sports medicine specialist at the Rothman Institute.
- Pramod Voleti, MD reviewed Disorders of the AC Joint and Bursitis of the Knee. Dr. Voleti is an orthopaedic surgeon and sports medicine specialist at the Albert Einstein College of Medicine.
- Miltiadis Zgonis, MD reviewed Disorders of the Glenoid Labrum. Dr. Zgonis is an orthopaedic surgeon and sports medicine specialist at the University of Pennsylvania.

The material was also reviewed by the following students from the Perelman School of Medicine at the University of Pennsylvania:

- Alexander Beschloss
- Joshua T. Bram
- Olivia G. Cohen
- Mitchell Johnson
- Ariana Meltzer-Bruhn
- Anchi B. Numfor
- Steven D. Tsai

A NECESSARY DISCLAIMER

Peer-review notwithstanding, this being 21st century America, we must include the following Disclaimer, similar to those found in works produced by well known authors and organizations.

This material was prepared for educational purposes only. We therefore disclaim any and all liability for any damages resulting to any individual which may arise out of the use of the material presented here. We similarly disclaim responsibility for any errors or omissions or for results obtained from the use of information contained here.

This material is not intended to represent the only, nor necessarily best, method or procedure appropriate for the medical situations discussed, but rather is intended to present an approach which may be helpful to others who face similar situations. We cannot can take any responsibility for the consequences following the application of any of the information presented here.

The information provided here cannot substitute for the advice of a medical professional. *Even if a given statement is completely true in the abstract, it may not apply to a given patient.*

The information we offer is provided "as is" and without warranty of any kind.

LIST OF CONTRIBUTORS

CONTRIBUTING EDITORS

The final version of this volume was produced by editing, refining and merging material from individual contributions as well as the material posted the OrthopaedicsOne wiki. The following authors listed below generously contributed to these raw chapters, and even more generously allowed their work to be edited, refined and merged (according to the overall needs of the project).

Richard Campbell	Thomas Hart	Nathaniel Mercer
Michele Caravella	Devan Higginbothamn	Trevor Ottofaro
Nicket Dedhia	Eoghan Hurley	Mili Parikh
Patrick Donaghue	David Ivanov	William Pham
Christopher Emerson	Zain Khazi	Sudah Suleimen
Ali Eternad-Rezaie	Dammy Kolade	Brian Thompson
Michael Fisher	Mark Lawlor	Joseph Tracey
Christopher Hadley	Christopher Lee	Brian Winters MD
Sommer Hammoud MD	Kevin Lutsky, MD	Barrett Woods MD

EDITORIAL ASSISTANCE

We are grateful for the expert editorial help provided by Megan Flinner, www.ManagedByMegan.com

PHOTOGRAPHY

We thank Paul Tjoumakaris and Deonde Degennaro, ATC for demonstrating the physical examination maneuvers.

COVER ART

Cover art designed and donated by:
Louis C. Okafor, MD
louisokafor@gmail.com

CHAPTER 1.

STRESS FRACTURES AND THE FEMALE ATHLETIC TRIAD

DESCRIPTION

The Female Athlete Triad was initially defined as the constellation of three interrelated clinical entities typically found in active young women: amenorrhea, osteoporosis, and disordered eating. The definition has now been broadened to recognize that each component of the triad exists on a spectrum. Thus, menstrual irregularities (without amenorrhea), low bone mineral density (without full-blown osteoporosis) and deficits of energy availability due to a deficient nutrition (without a formal diagnosis of an eating disorder) may be sufficient to prompt this diagnosis. Notably, the Triad can appear when there is not enough caloric intake to balance caloric expenditure, independent of whether that imbalance is intentional or unintentional. For example, many runners do not realize how much to increase intake as they ramp up their training.

The Female Athlete Triad can have significant medical ramifications outside of musculoskeletal medicine – notably gynecological and psychological. Patients with the Female Athlete Triad usually come to attention of musculoskeletal practitioners because of stress fractures: skeletal damage caused by repetitive loading forces that exceed the bone's mechanical resiliency.

The Female Athlete Triad is also relevant to musculoskeletal medicine in that even without a stress fracture, patients with this condition may fail to attain an optimal peak bone mass in adolescence –the time of maximal bone formation– and thus place themselves at higher risk for osteoporosis later in life.

STRUCTURE AND FUNCTION

Female athletes, especially those who participate in an activity that values a thin physique, may choose to eat too little or exercise too much. In the extreme, some may starve themselves (anorexia nervosa) or overeat and purge (bulimia).

Insufficient nutrition has two important consequences for bone health. For one thing, a calcium deficiency may be present. Also, decreased body fat is associated with decreased estrogen levels as well. Low estrogen can be recognized by amenorrhea, but its deficiency can also cause clinically silent damage to the bone. Estrogen is a potent mediator of both osteoclast and osteoblast activity. Without appropriate levels of this hormone, bone remodeling is disrupted.

Bone remodeling is the process that repairs the (micro)damage induced by regular activity. It also adjusts the bone's architecture to better withstand the mechanical stresses placed on it.

Remodeling is achieved through the coupled action of osteoclasts and osteoblasts. Osteoclasts resorb bone, and osteoblasts synthesize new bone matrix which then becomes mineralized.

Activities that apply cyclic loading forces can lead to the formation of microfractures. (Running is the prototypical "cyclic loading forces" activity but not the only one; rowing and throwing are commonly seen causes as well.) When the rate of damage accumulation becomes greater than the rate of remodeling, these microfractures can lengthen and coalesce, resulting in a stress fracture.

PATIENT PRESENTATION

Patients with stress fractures will classically present with insidious onset of pain that acutely worsens with high impact activity and improves with rest. Pain onset is often several weeks after a notable increase in a familiar physical activity and is not associated with a specific injury. For example, a runner who recently increased her training from 5 to 10 miles per day may present with new symptoms.

Any female athlete who presents with a stress fracture should be questioned for the presence of factors associated with the Female Athlete Triad. The patient should first be asked about activities and nutrition. As a first approximation, athletes should eat about 45 kCal per Kg of lean body mass, in addition to the sports-specific energy demands (e.g., approximately 100 kCal for every mile ran). In addition, they should be asked about their menstrual history and use of birth control pills. A history of prior stress fractures, weight changes or other diseases that may affect bone health (e.g., thyroid disease) should also be reviewed.

The first physical finding to assess is the body mass index (BMI). BMI is defined as the body mass divided by the square of the body height. Because self-reporting is imprecise, formal measurement should be made. According to the 2014 Female Athlete Triad Coalition Consensus Statement, a BMI below 18.5 kg/m^2 represents moderate risk and a BMI below 17.5 kg/m^2 is high risk.

On physical exam, stress fractures often have no objective findings at all. Point tenderness or swelling may or may not be present. If there is a high index of suspicion, a thorough exam of the implicated bone is warranted. The 3-point fulcrum test is useful in identifying femoral shaft stress fractures and is considered positive if pain is elicited. Additionally, a calcaneal squeeze test that elicits pain can indicate a calcaneal stress fracture of the foot (See Figure 1).

Figure 1: Squeezing calcaneus side to side may reveal a stress fracture.

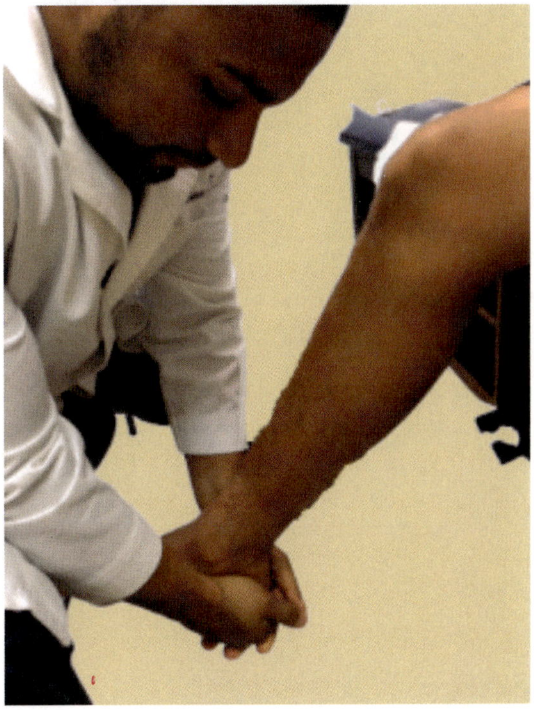

Soft, thin hair on the extremities (so-called "lanugo"), scarred knuckles, and parotid gland enlargement are physical exam findings seen in patients with anorexia or bulimia nervosa. Bradycardia and low blood pressure can be signs of malnutrition or low energy availability, but this is difficult to differentiate from a physically fit athlete with a slow baseline resting heart rate.

OBJECTIVE EVIDENCE

In Female Athlete Triad, each of the three components can be assessed independently, which can help guide treatment. In low energy availability states, electrolyte abnormalities such as hypokalemia, hyponatremia, or an acid-base disturbance may be present.

Menstrual disturbances should first be assessed with a urine pregnancy test. Other lab values can provide insight on the functioning of the hypothalamic pituitary adrenal axis including luteinizing hormone (LH) and follicle-stimulating hormone, prolactin, and thyroid stimulating hormone (TSH).

Assessing bone mineral density with dual-energy x-ray absorptiometry (DEXA) is critically important for patients with Female Athlete Triad, especially if she has already had a stress fracture. A Z-score less than +1.0 in a young athlete should prompt further evaluation because bone mineral density is expected to be higher in those who regularly participate in weight-bearing activity.

Typically, patients with stress fractures will have normal radiographic findings. Positive findings are more likely to be found several weeks after symptom onset. These findings include cortical radiolucency, periosteal reaction (see Figure 2), endosteal or cortical thickening, and (in the rare case) a fracture line.

Figure 2: Stress fracture of 2nd metatarsal identified by the surrounding periosteal reaction. (Case courtesy of Dr. Vikas Shah, rID 62575, Radiopaedia.org)

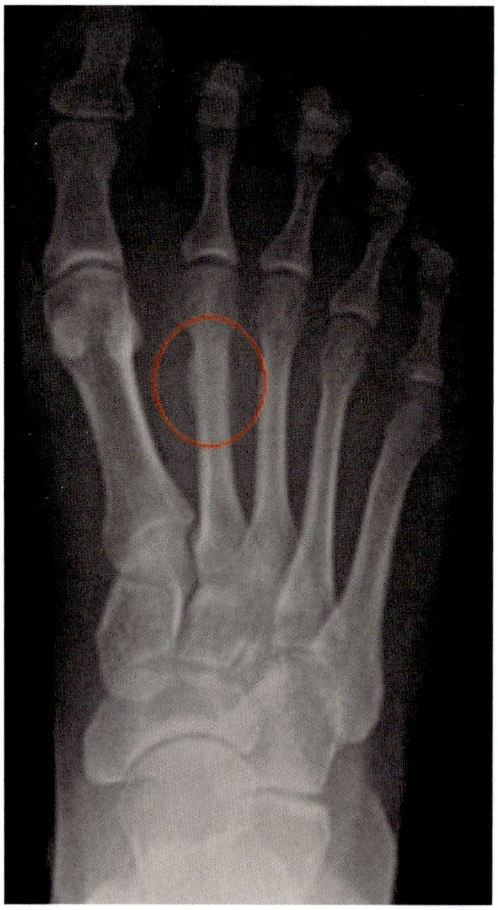

MRI and technetium bone scans are the best diagnostic imaging tests for identifying occult stress fractures (see Figure 3). T1 and T2-weighted MRIs will pick up marrow edema and delineate clear fracture lines. Tc99m bone scan will show focal uptake at the stress fracture site.

Figure 3: Stress fracture of distal tibia. Radiograph on left shows a subtle area of sclerosis whereas the T1-weighted MRI on the right clearly demonstrates the incomplete fracture line at the distal tibial metaphysis. (Case courtesy of Dr. Hani Salam, rID 8720, Radiopaedia.org)

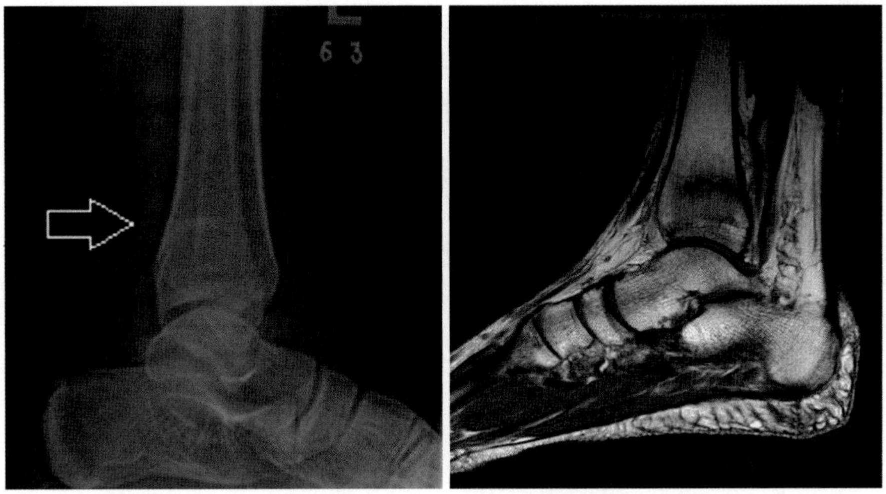

Figure 4: Calcaneal stress fracture. A nuclear bone scan shows tracer uptake at the stress fracture location. (Case courtesy of Radswiki, Radiopaedia.org, rID: 11969)

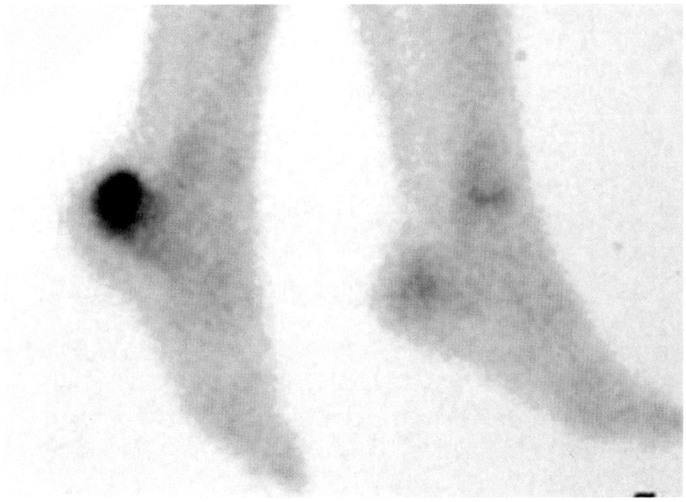

EPIDEMIOLOGY

Female Athlete Triad is most commonly seen in adolescents and young adults. Sports in which a thin figure and light weight are competitively advantageous, such as ballet, cheerleading, gymnastics, and cross-country running, are often implicated. Athletes of any sport can develop the condition.

According to the American Academy of Pediatrics, it is difficult to estimate the true prevalence of the triad as each of the components may be expressed in varying severity. Moreover, not all components are present simultaneously. Beyond that, prevalence is assessed by self-reported (and possibly imprecise) metrics in cross-sectional studies. With that caveat, the frequently used approximation is that 1% of high school athletes have all three components and that the prevalence of at least one component may be as high 50%.

It is also difficult to estimate the true prevalence of stress fractures, primarily because many cases do not present for medical attention. Also, among those fractures that are seen, treatment (in the form of relative rest) is often initiated empirically without objective confirmation. Stress fractures are most commonly seen in weight bearing bones of the leg (e.g. the metatarsals and calcaneus most commonly). They can also occur in the tibia, fibula, navicular, femur and bones of the upper body. Young military recruits are another population where stress fractures are commonly identified, especially within the first several months of their training. In this population these injuries are often called "March Fractures," and classically occur in the 2nd metatarsal.

DIFFERENTIAL DIAGNOSIS

Lower extremity pain in an athlete without a history of overt injury suggests the diagnosis of stress fracture, but this may also be the presentation of a simple muscle strain. Pain that does not get better with rest may suggest more serious conditions such as bone tumors or infection. Radiographs in patients with suspicious symptoms are essential. Because the x-ray presentation of stress fractures, tumors, and infections can be similar, MRI or other advanced testing may be needed as well.

RED FLAGS

A diagnosis of Female Athlete Triad should be high on the differential when any of the following are present:

- Any female athlete that presents with a stress fracture,
- Body mass index below 20,
- Oligomenorrhea or amenorrhea in a competitive athlete,
- Concerning comments about weight gain, weight loss, calorie restriction, or body image.

There should be a high index of suspicion for a stress fracture when any of the following are present:

- An athlete who presents with pain in the lower extremity without a clear history of an injury,
- History of dramatic increase in a specific physical activity,
- Acutely worsening and localizing pain with exercise and significant relief with rest.

The Female Athlete Triad is itself a "red-flag" for the presence of other conditions that may be beyond the expertise of a musculoskeletal medicine specialist. These include gynecological abnormalities, endocrine disorders (e.g. polycystic ovary syndrome, hyper/hypothyroidism), complications of pharmaceuticals (both prescribed and illicit), and psychological disorders. It is critical to make the appropriate referral to a provider with the relevant expertise.

Stress fracture of the superior femoral neck (the so-called "tension side" of the neck) can propagate and displace the femoral head from the shaft. (This contrasts with such fractures on the inferior neck, the "compression side" (see Figure 5), which, should they propagate, will collapse upon themselves.) In turn, such displacement may disrupt the blood supply to the femoral head and cause osteonecrosis. This is a rare complication of a rare condition, but the consequences of missing it can be catastrophic. Thus, a presentation suggesting a stress fracture of the hip demands diligent attention, prompt imaging and referral to an orthopaedic surgeon if the diagnosis is confirmed.

Figure 5: MRI showing stress fracture of the inferior femoral neck with surrounding edema. (Courtesy of https://radiopaedia.org/cases/femoral-neck-stress-fracture-3)

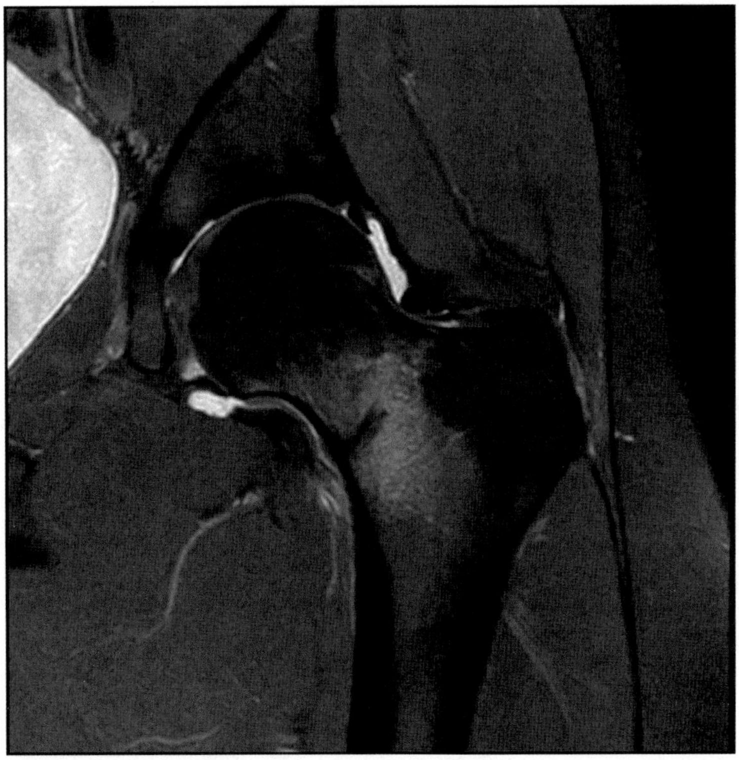

TREATMENT OPTIONS AND OUTCOMES

The primary goal in treating Female Athlete Triad is restoring energy balance, which will help restore menstrual regularity and improve bone mineral density. Nutrition education, modifying diet and physical activity, and partnering with mental health services are important methods in treating energy availability.

Calcium and vitamin D supplementations are also important in restoring bone health. Contrary to recommendations for the older population, bisphosphonates are not recommended in treating low bone mineral density or osteoporosis in patients with Female Athlete Triad, as their use increases the risk of stress fractures.

The treatment goal for Female Athlete Triad is restoring energy balance and improving bone mineral density. Clinical success can be gauged by weight gain and resumption of menses. Screening and early diagnosis of this condition is essential as bone loss during adolescence and early adulthood is not recoverable and impacts the patient's peak bone mineral density later in life.

The mainstay of treatment of stress fractures is rest and avoidance. Activity is restricted, and athletes cannot return to play until pain subsides, tenderness has resolved, and radiographic findings are negative.

Stress fractures of metatarsals, femoral shaft, and tibial shaft can generally be managed with modified weight bearing. Fractures in the calcaneus and navicular may require a stricter non-weight bearing status.

Open reduction and internal fixation (ORIF) may be considered in elite or professional athletes who require a faster recovery and are at high risk of complications, such as displacement or nonunion.

Operative treatment is also indicated for fractures in locations at high risk of fracture propagation or poor healing, such as on the tension side of the femoral neck or on the anterior cortex of tibia. Surgery is also indicated when non-operative measures have failed.

Persistent weight bearing on a stress fracture may cause arrest of bone healing or lead to a complete fracture, increasing the risk of displacement and nonunion. Stress fractures have an overall excellent prognosis when treated appropriately (operative vs non-operative, non-weight bearing vs modified weight bearing) and the patient is educated on physical activity modification.

RISK FACTORS AND PREVENTION

Participation in sports that place value on thinness, either for esthetic reasons (e.g. gymnastics) or performance (e.g. long-distance running) may increase the risk of developing the Female Athlete Triad. Another risk factor is playing a sport in which athletes compete in weight divisions (e.g. light-weight rowing).

Lack of nutritional education in a competitive athlete is also a known risk factor.

Prevention of the Female Athlete Triad may be helped by screening and early recognition. Screening can be accomplished during sports physicals with questionnaires or through targeted history-taking. Information such as menstrual history, dietary habits, body image assessment, and eating behaviors can identify females at risk and aid in the diagnosis if Female Athlete Triad is already present.

Athletes with a sudden increase in their level of activity are at risk for stress fracture: the process of bone remodeling is overwhelmed. This can be mitigated by well-conceived training schedule.

MISCELLANY

The Female Athlete Triad is typically not denoted by the acronym FAT–perhaps because the syndrome is characterized by a lack of fat.

KEY TERMS

Female Athlete Triad, stress fractures, low energy availability, amenorrhea, bone mineral density, osteoporosis, insufficiency fractures, march fractures, bone remodeling

SKILLS

Identify athletes at risk of Female Athlete Triad. Obtain the relevant history in a respectful manner likely to elicit complete information. Recognize the signs, symptoms and radiographic findings of stress fracture. Educate the patient on activity modification and strategies to prevent future stress fractures.

CHAPTER 2.

BURNERS AND STINGERS

DESCRIPTION

A burner or stinger is characterized by brief, unilateral arm pain, paresthesias or weakness after an injury or a specific inciting event. A burner or stinger is caused by a transient brachial plexus injury (so-called neuropraxia) due to traction, compression, or direct trauma to the brachial plexus. It is often associated with collision sports injuries, such as football, that causes bending of the neck and/or displacement of the arm. Treatment is usually not necessary, and players can return to play when and if there is complete resolution of symptoms.

STRUCTURE AND FUNCTION

The brachial plexus comprises of nerve roots from C5-T1 (Figure 1). There are five regions to the brachial plexus from proximal to distal: Roots, Trunks, Divisions, Cords, Branches.

Figure 1: A "wiring diagram" of the brachial plexus. (from https://en.wikipedia.org/wiki/Brachial_plexus)

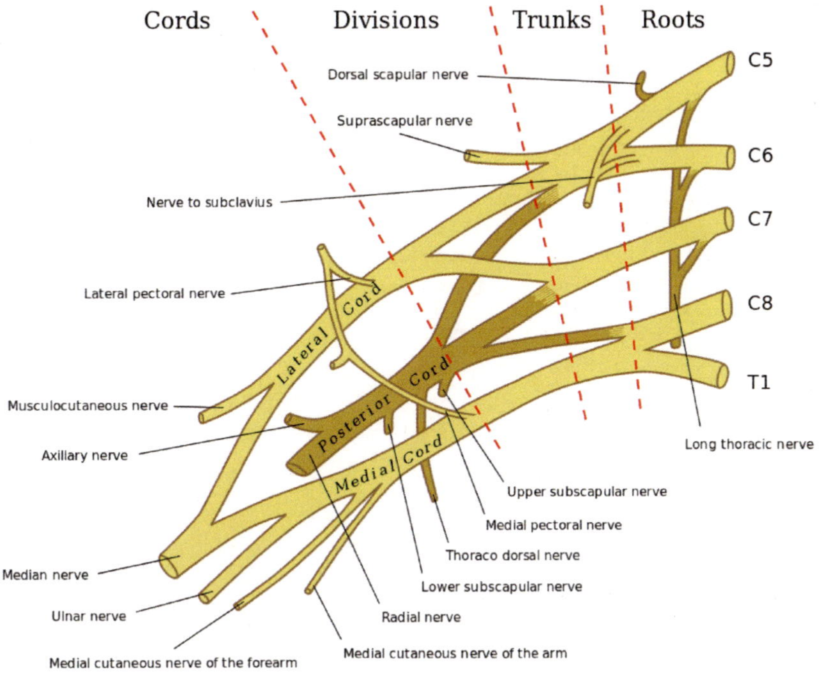

Roots – The nerve roots are composed of the ventral and dorsal components, each carrying motor and sensory information, respectively. The two combine to form the cervical nerve roots and exit the spine. The 5 cervical roots combine to form 3 trunks.

Trunks – The superior (C5, C6), middle (C7), and inferior (C8, T1) trunks emerge between the anatomical triangle formed by the anterior scalene muscle, middle scalene muscle, and the first rib. After traversing a short distance, each trunk divides into anterior and posterior divisions.

Divisions – There are six divisions (3 anterior, 3 posterior) that combine into 3 cords, which now have different coverage from the C5-T1 roots compared to the 3 trunks.

Cords – The posterior cord (C5-C8) is formed from the 3 posterior divisions. Prior to the final branches, the posterior cord gives off the upper subscapular nerve (C5, C6; innervates subscapularis), the lower subscapular nerve (C5, C6; innervates subscapularis and teres major), and the thoracodorsal nerve (C6-C8; innervates latissimus dorsi).

The lateral cord (C5-C7) is formed from the anterior divisions of the superior and middle trunks. Prior to its final branching, it gives off the lateral pectoral nerve (C5-C7; innervates pectoralis major).

The medial cord (C8, T1) is formed from the anterior division of the inferior trunk. Prior to its final branching, it gives off the medial pectoral nerve (C8, T1; innervates pectoralis minor and major), the medial brachial cutaneous nerve (T1), and the medial antebrachial cutaneous nerve (C8, T1). Each cord gives off two terminal branches.

Branches – There are five terminal branches (two branches form the median nerve).

1. The axillary nerve (C5, C6) derives from the posterior cord and travels to the glenohumeral joint. It mainly innervates the deltoid as well as sensation to the lateral shoulder.
2. The radial nerve (C5-T1) derives from the posterior cord and runs medially along the arm with the long head of the triceps until it crosses laterally across the humerus via the spiral groove. The nerve supplies the elbow and forearm extensors and supinators. The nerve also provides sensation to the distal-lateral arm, the posterior forearm, and the posterior aspect of the radial side of the hand (thumb to middle finger).
3. The median nerve (C5-C7) derives from the medial and the lateral cord. The cords join anterior to the axillary artery and then travels with the artery along the arm. The nerve innervates most wrist flexors and pronators as well as the two lumbricals on the radial side of the hand. The nerve provides sensation to the anterior aspect of the radial side of the hand.
4. The musculocutaneous nerve (C5-C7) derives from the medial cord and pierces through the coracobrachialis muscle to become the most superficial branch. The nerve innervates the biceps, coracobrachialis, and brachialis. The nerve provides sensation to the lateral forearm.
5. The ulnar nerve (C8, T1) derives from the medial cord and runs along the medial aspect of the arm, through the cubital tunnel at the elbow and through Guyon's canal at the wrist. The nerve innervates the flexor carpi ulnaris, the adductor pollicis, and the intrinsic hand muscles (except the two radial lumbricals innervated by the median nerve). The nerve provides sensation to the whole ulnar aspect of the hand.

Most cases of stingers affect the C5/C6 nerve roots or the upper trunk of the plexus.

The most common cause of injury is due to traction on the brachial plexus rather than direct trauma. This can occur in ipsilateral shoulder depression and neck deviation towards the contralateral side, often seen in tackling, which causes stretching of the brachial plexus on the ipsilateral side.

PATIENT PRESENTATION

Most athletes present after particularly high-impact collisions, with immediate onset of unilateral, radiating, and severe burning pain down the arm. This may be accompanied by paresthesia in the related sensory dermatome (the area of skin sensation supplied by a given spinal nerve) and motor weakness. Players may be supporting the affected arm using the other arm to relieve tension. Neck pain is usually not present.

On physical exam, transient sensory disturbances (numbness, tingling, burning, or radiating pain) in the affected arm are common (Figure 2). There may be transient, unilateral weakness in the affected arm with normal biceps reflexes (Figure 3 – Figure 7). (Transient hyporeflexia may be present in a minority of patients).

Figure 2: The sensory dermatomes as shown on the volar (palmar) side of the arm. Lesions at the given level would be expected to produce sensory changes in these locations, if any.

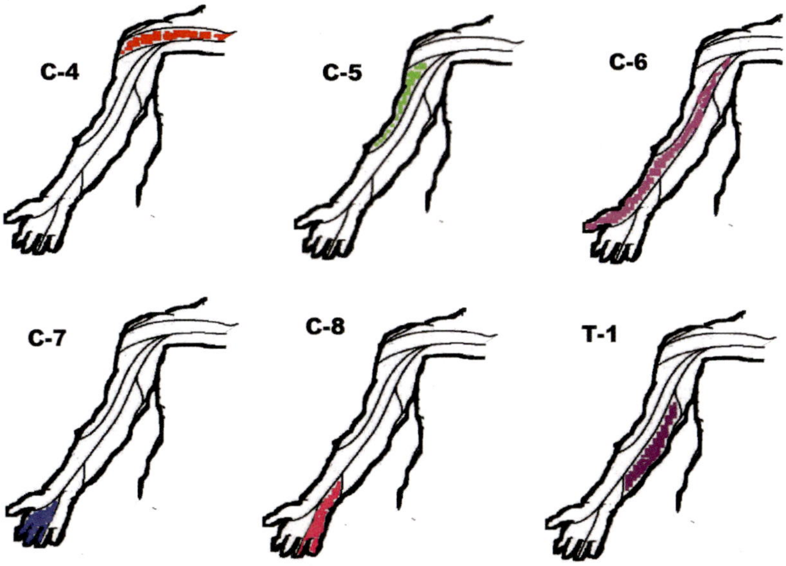

Figure 3: C-5 Motor exam: assessing shoulder abduction. With the elbow flexed, the patient abducts the shoulder to 90. The examiner pushes down on the elbow as the patient resists with deltoid activity.

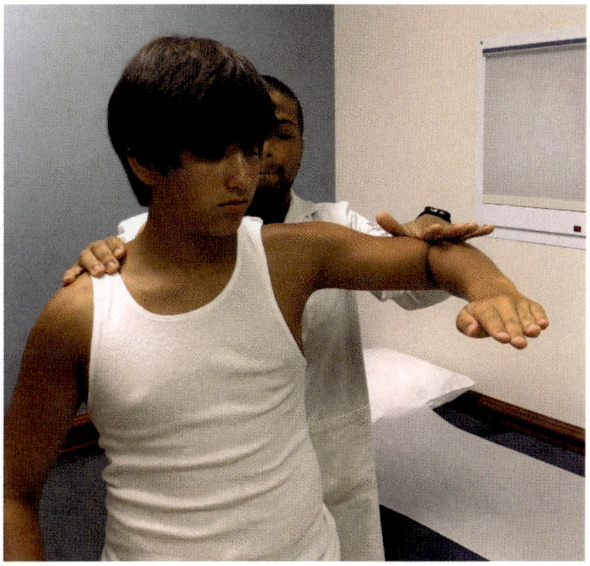

Figure 4: The C-6 Motor exam: assessing wrist extension. With the forearm pronated, the patient extends the wrist. The examiner can assess strength by pushing down on the knuckle of the index finger as the patient resists with radial wrist extensor activity.

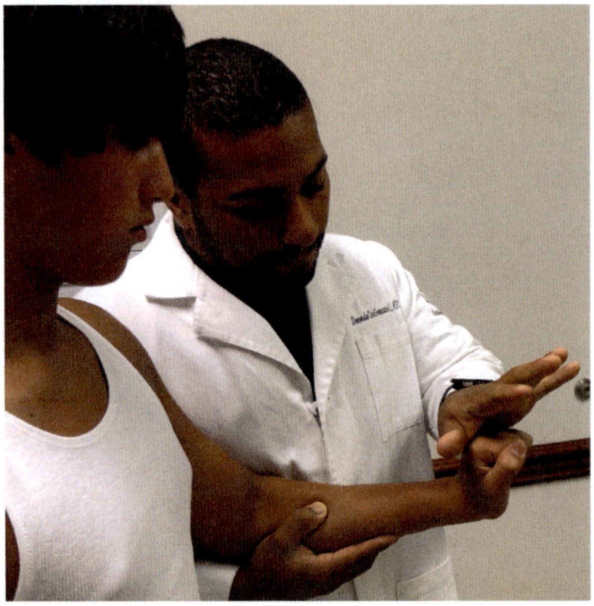

Figure 5: The C-7 Motor exam: assessing wrist flexion. With fingers extended, the patient flexes the wrist. The examiner pushes against the palm to force the wrist into extension as the patient resists. (As with the C-6 exam, the patient's fingers are positioned to eliminate the indirect effect of finger muscles on wrist motion.)

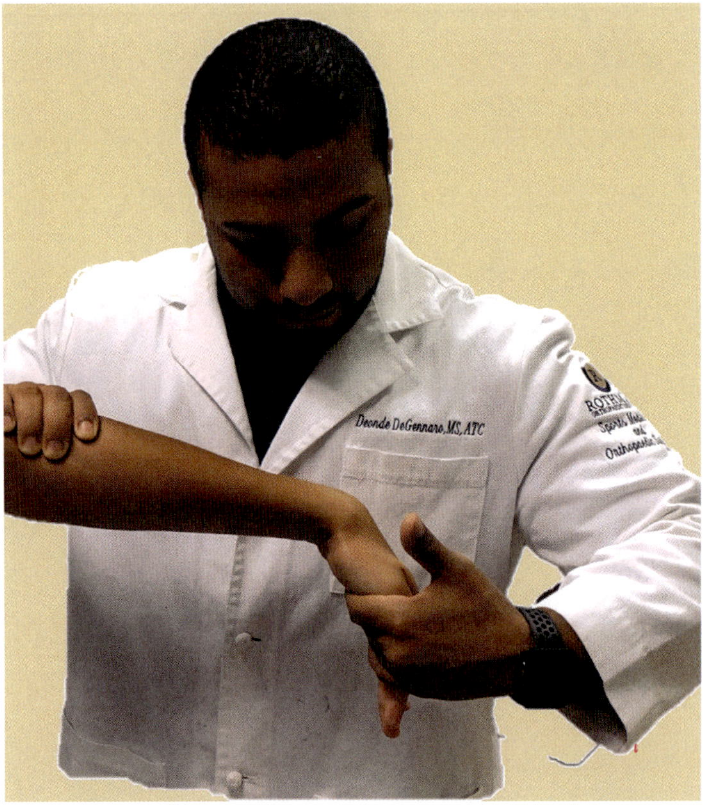

Figure 6: The C-8 Motor exam: assessing finger flexion/grip strength. Have the patient attempt to squeeze the examiner's index and long finger simultaneously.

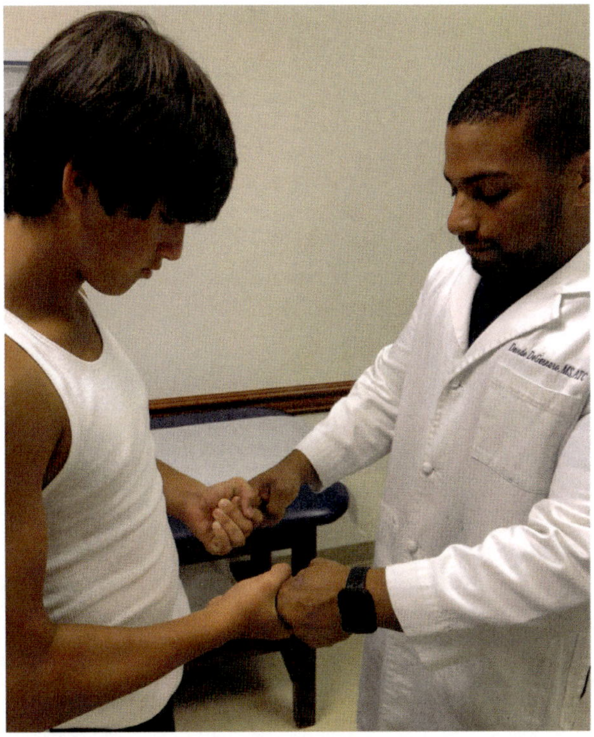

Figure 7: The T-1 Motor examination: assessing finger abduction. Ask the patient to spread (abduct) the fingers and hold that position; the examiner can assess strength by attempting to resist this as shown.

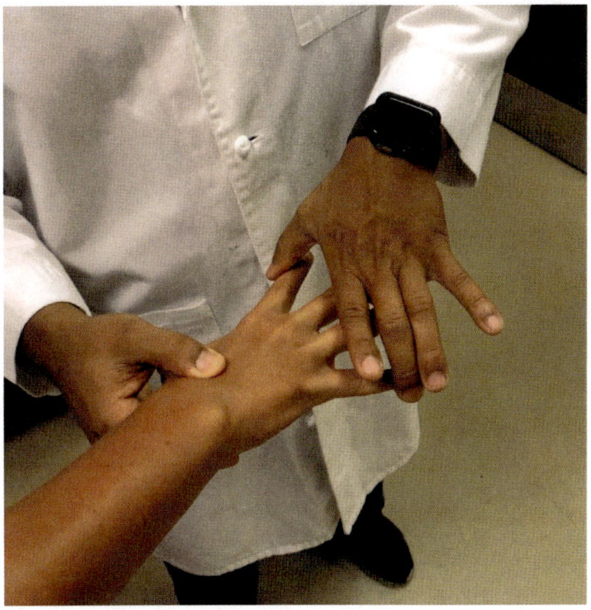

The lower extremity exam should be normal, and if it is not, the diagnosis of a stinger is questioned.

The key finding is that these symptoms, if present, should be transient. The vast majority of cases resolve within a few minutes to days.

All cases of stingers can be classified into 3 grades. Grade 1 stingers are due to neuropraxia (intact axon but demyelinated). There may be temporary loss of sensation and/or motor function up to days. Grade 2 stingers are due to axonotmesis (axon damage). This produces more significant motor and/or sensory deficits which may last up to several weeks. Last, Grade 3 stingers are due to neurotmesis (severed nerves). This may produce enduring symptoms that may never fully resolve.

OBJECTIVE EVIDENCE

In most cases of first-time stingers, imaging is not necessary. Initial imaging, if obtained, usually consists of anterior-posterior, lateral, and oblique views of the cervical spine and shoulder area. No abnormal findings are found in most cases of simple stingers. If there are concerns for further pathology due to Red Flag findings mentioned below, and if initial imaging is normal, cervical MRI should be obtained to evaluate the spinal cord, nerve roots, vertebral discs, ligamentous injury, or vertebral fractures.

There are no specific laboratory findings associated with stingers or other cervical spine diseases.

EPIDEMIOLOGY

Stingers are most commonly seen in football players, but can also be seen in hockey, lacrosse, and rugby players. This is because the mechanism of injury is usually forced rapid lateral neck flexion, which can occur during tackling and can cause traction or compression injuries to the brachial plexus. It is estimated that over 50% of football players have reported at least one stinger during their career. The true prevalence of this condition is not known, mainly due to its transient nature and the tendency of players to not report or underreport their symptoms.

DIFFERENTIAL DIAGNOSIS

The differential diagnosis for stingers is relatively narrow but should be considered in any cases when red flags (as discussed below) are present.

- Cervical radiculopathy: Consider if symptoms persist beyond 24 hours. MRI can help assess for radiculopathy. Presentation may be similar to burners and stingers, other than the timeframe of symptoms.
- Shoulder dislocation or acromioclavicular joint injury: Injury to the bony structures of the shoulder should be considered, especially after traumatic sports injuries affecting one arm. X-rays, CT, or MRI can help assess for injuries to the bones or surrounding soft tissue.
- Thoracic outlet syndrome: This syndrome is thought to be caused by compression of the brachial plexus or subclavian vessels as they pass through narrow passageways leading from the base of the neck and torso out to the arm (the "thoracic outlet"). This compression can cause neck and arm pain and paresthesias in the fingers and hand. At times, the affected hand is pale and cool. Thoracic outlet syndrome seems to be provoked by rotation of the head and neck.
- Cervical spine stenosis or fracture: In severe cases of collision, the actual spinal canal may be damaged. If this is the case, players may present with bilateral symptoms or have symptoms in their lower extremities, which never occurs with stingers. The cervical spine should be immobilized until further evaluation by CT or MRI.

RED FLAGS

If any of the following signs are present in a patient presenting for stingers, further workup should be considered to rule out the above differential diagnoses.

- Bilateral symptoms: Stingers affect only one arm at a time. Bilateral symptoms should raise concern for spinal canal stenosis or cervical fractures.
- Lower extremity symptoms: Stingers affect only the brachial plexus. Lower extremity symptoms should raise concern for spinal cord injuries.
- Muscle atrophy: Stingers, due to their transient nature, rarely causes atrophy. If significant atrophy is present, consider recurrent stingers or other pathologies.
- Symptoms lasting more than 24 hours: While stingers can last longer than 24 hours, the majority of cases last under 24 hours. Further imaging should be pursued if symptoms last for over 24 hours to rule out more dangerous pathologies, covered above.

TREATMENT OPTIONS AND OUTCOMES

The most important step in treating suspected stingers is to remove the player from play for initial evaluation. A quick but thorough exam of all four extremities as well as the neck should be conducted to assess for findings and red flags discussed in this chapter. A player may return to play upon complete resolution of symptoms and once he/she demonstrates normal strength and range of motion of the affected arm. Recurring or persistent symptoms should be evaluated as discussed earlier. If symptoms last for more than a few minutes, cervical x-rays should be strongly considered to evaluate for fractures or dislocations.

For persistent symptoms, after appropriate work up showing no other pathology, rest and gentle stretching of the affected arm is advised. Physical therapy may be recommended if symptoms persist beyond a few days. Specific stretching and posturing maneuvers can be recommended by the therapist. NSAIDs may be used to alleviate pain during the first few days.

Surgery is almost never considered for stingers. In rare cases of Grade 3 stingers, due to complete transection of axons, surgery may be attempted to repair the damaged axons, but outcomes are poor.

Considering that stingers rarely lead to permanent disability, the general prognosis of first-time stingers is excellent. An estimated 85% players are able to return to play within the same game or practice. A history of a prior stinger can increase the incidence of recurrent stingers, but there is no clear evidence of recurrent stingers causing permanent nerve injury.

RISK FACTORS AND PREVENTION

The most significant risk factor for the development of stingers is playing contact sports that involve tackling. The majority of such players encounter at least one episode of stingers during their career. The presence of cervical canal stenosis has been associated with increased risk of stingers in athletes.

Prevention efforts should focus on proper tackling techniques and protective equipment. A more upright tackling position may protect the neck from excessive extension, while increased padding and/or cervical collar may help absorb some of the impact.

MISCELLANY

The five sections of the brachial plexus, in order from proximal to distal (roots, trunks, divisions, cords, branches), can be memorized by the following mnemonic (Randy Travis Drinks Cold Beer).

The three terminal branches that form the famous M of the brachial plexus, in order from lateral to medial (musculocutaneous, median, ulnar), can be recalled by thinking MuMU (μ, M in Greek).

KEY TERMS

Cervical spine, brachial plexus, stingers/burners, sensory dermatome

SKILLS

Draw a "wiring diagram" of the brachial plexus from memory. (It's always on the test!) Perform a comprehensive physical exam to evaluate neurologic signs and symptoms. Counsel players on safe sports techniques and appropriate equipment to reduce future recurrences.

CHAPTER 3.

SPONDYLOLYSIS AND SPONDYLOLISTHESIS

DESCRIPTION

Spondylolysis and spondylolisthesis are relatively common causes of low back pain, especially in young athletes. Spondylolysis refers to a weakening or other defect in a specific region of the vertebra called the pars interarticularis. These defects may be caused by repetitive stress. Spondylolisthesis refers to anterior slippage (displacement) of the vertebrae. This is often the result of bilateral spondylolysis, a so-called isthmic spondylolisthesis. Thus, spondylolysis and spondylolisthesis are separate yet interrelated conditions.

Besides isthmic spondylolisthesis, there are several other notable subtypes of spondylolisthesis. The two other most common forms are degenerative spondylolisthesis and dysplastic (congenital) spondylolisthesis. Less common forms include traumatic, pathologic, and iatrogenic/post-surgical.

STRUCTURE AND FUNCTION

The human spine has 24 vertebrae stacked one on top of the other: seven cervical, twelve thoracic and five lumbar. The lowest lumbar vertebra, L5, sits atop the sacrum. The vertebral bodies are separated by intervertebral discs, which function both as elastic bearings permitting motion as well as shock absorbers dissipating forces transmitted through the spinal column.

Behind the vertebral body lie the so-called posterior elements of the spine: the pedicles, the lamina and three processes: the transverse, the articular, and the spinous processes (Figure 1). The posterior elements connect to the vertebral body via the pedicles. At the dorsal limit of the pedicle is the pars interarticularis. The pars then extends cephalad to become the superior articular process and caudad to become the inferior articular process. The transverse process projects laterally from the pars in the thoracic and lumbar spine. Coursing dorsally from the pars, the laminae extend dorsally and medially to connect in the midline and complete the ring around the spinal canal. The spinous process is a dorsal extension from the junction of the two laminae at the midline.

Figure 1: Schematic drawings of a lumbar vertebra, seen from above (axial view, on the left) and from the side (lateral view, right). VB: vertebral body; TP: transverse process (omitted from drawing on the right as it projects out of the plane); SP: spinous process. As seen from above, the central canal, behind the vertebral body, is surrounded by the pedicles (red), lamina (purple) and the superior and inferior articulating processes and the bone that connects them, the pars intraarticularis (gray).

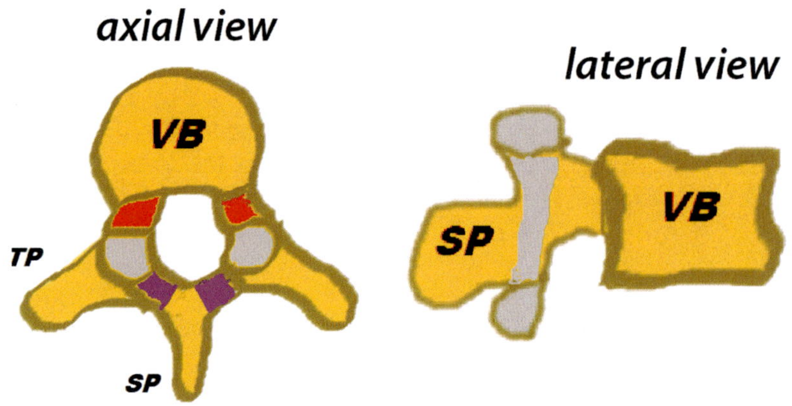

Damage to the pars can incite an attempt at healing. The resultant hypertrophic fibrous tissue can cause foraminal stenosis with compression of the exiting nerve root. This most commonly occurs at L5-S1, resulting in an L5 radiculopathy.

On each side, left and right, the inferior articular processes of the vertebra above and the superior articular processes of the vertebra below, come together to form the facet joints. The function of the facet joint is to guide and also limit motion of the spine. Specifically, the facet joints in the lumbar spine permit flexion, extension, and rotation while simultaneously preventing extremes of these motions as well as translation.

Because the pars bridges the articular processes to the vertebral body, damage to the pars results in functional incompetence of the facet joints. It is this loss of restraint that allows anterior displacement or "slippage" of the superior vertebral body: spondylolisthesis (Figure 2).

Figure 2: If there is a pars defect, the bodies above can slip forward relative to the body below.

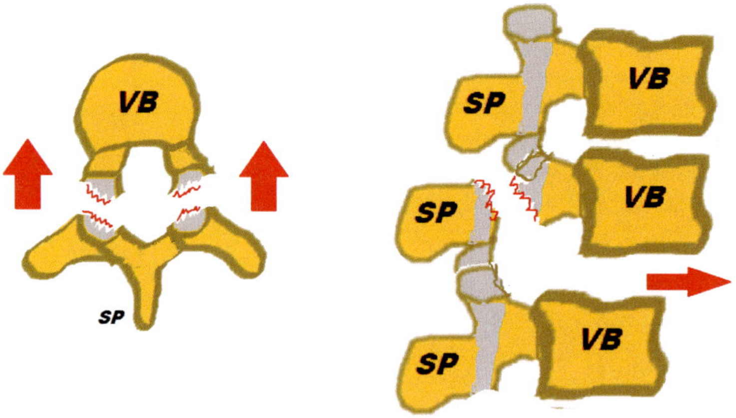

In the vast majority of cases, spondylolysis is a developmental defect that may be present in up to 5-7 percent of the population and is typically asymptomatic. In the setting of new onset low back pain, spondylolysis may occur from overuse causing microfracture. In rare circumstances, a fracture in the pars articularis can occur following an acute load or trauma.

While the progression from a pars defect to spondylolisthesis is the mechanism of isthmic type spondylolisthesis, the pathophysiology of degenerative spondylolisthesis is different. In the most fundamental sense, the major difference between isthmic and degenerative forms is the *absence* of a defect in the pars interarticularis causing the anterior displacement in degenerative spondylolisthesis. Instead, the pathophysiology in degenerative spondylolisthesis centers around degeneration of the facet joint and intervertebral discs, leading to instability and increased motion of the vertebra. Degenerative spondylolisthesis is most commonly seen at L4-L5. Because the pars remains intact, the posterior elements of the sliding vertebra must also slide as a unit. Thus, degenerative spondylolisthesis is more likely to result in stenosis within the canal (especially the subarticular region) affecting the traversing roots. This contrasts with the isolated foraminal stenosis typically encountered with isthmic spondylolisthesis.

With respect to the other, rarer forms of spondylolisthesis, the dysplastic (congenital) type occurs secondary to abnormal spine development in utero, traumatic is the result of severe traumatic injury leading to vertebral displacement, and pathologic refers to the presence of a secondary disease process resulting in instability and displacement of the vertebra, including osteoporosis, malignancy, or infection.

PATIENT PRESENTATION

The diagnosis of spondylolysis is often an incidental discovery on an x-ray without any clinical signs or symptoms. In fact, the majority of patients with radiographic evidence of spondylolysis are asymptomatic.

In patients with spondylolysis that have symptoms, however, the most common complaint is low back pain of gradual onset that is worsened with activity, especially activities which involve hyperextension of the lumbar spine. The quality of the pain is non-specific and may resemble that of an ordinary lumbar muscle strain.

The presentation of isthmic spondylolisthesis is similar to that of spondylolysis, with non-specific low back pain often being the primary complaint. In spondylolisthesis, however, there is a higher occurrence of radicular symptoms. Impingement of the L5 nerve root in the foramen is most common, resulting in radiculopathy (paresthesias or pain radiating to the legs, or "sciatica").

In rare circumstances, patients with spondylolisthesis can experience a "*listhetic* crisis" characterized by severe back pain, neurologic deficits, and hamstring spasm, all which may be exacerbated by extension of the lumbar spine.

On physical examination of patients with spondylolysis and spondylolisthesis, there may be evidence of increased lumbar lordosis (inward curvature of the spine), decreased range of motion of the spine, pain upon lumbar spine extension, or a palpable step off of the spinous process (representing anterior displacement in spondylolisthesis). They may also have sensory or motor findings on neurologic exam depending upon any underlying neural compression.

In degenerative spondylolisthesis, low back pain is the most common symptom as well. These patients, however, may experience neurogenic claudication and leg pain secondary to spinal canal stenosis, which is more common in the degenerative than the isthmic form.

OBJECTIVE EVIDENCE

The gold standard modality for the diagnosis of spondylolysis and spondylolisthesis are plain radiographs of the lumbar spine. The important views are standing anterior-posterior (AP) and lateral in the standing position. Oblique views may also be obtained, but these are unnecessary in most cases.

In the AP view, sclerosis of the pars interarticularis may be appreciated secondary to stress reaction. From the lateral view, a defect in the pars interarticularis is identifiable in the majority of cases (Figure 3).

Figure 3: A pars defect is shown in the red circle; a normal pars is seen above in the green circle. (Case courtesy of Radswiki, Radiopaedia.org, rID: 11967)

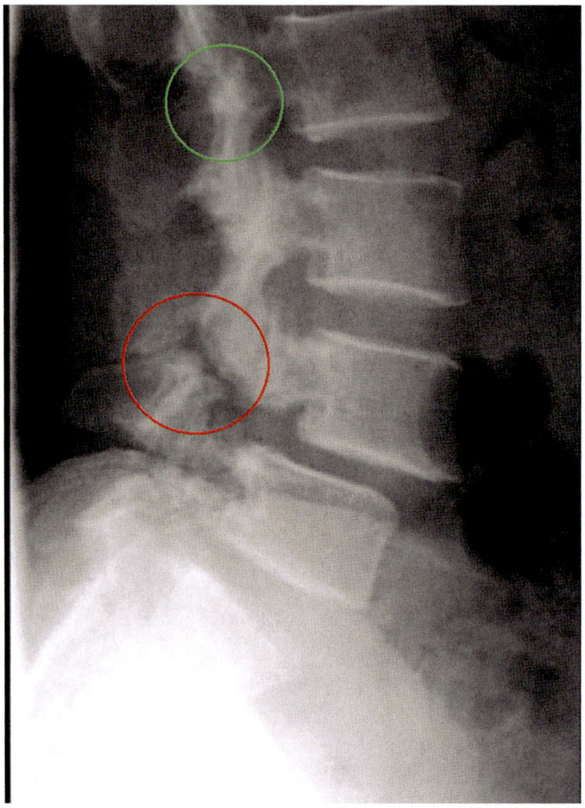

The oblique film is a more specific view in the assessment of spondylolysis and spondylolisthesis. From this angle, the vertebra in the lumbar spine demonstrate the classic "Scottie dog" appearance (Figure 4), consisting of the superior articular process (ears of the dog), transverse process (head), isthmus (neck), lamina and spinous process (body), and inferior articular processes (foreleg and hindleg). In spondylolysis, the defect in the pars interarticularis appears as a neck collar on the Scottie dog.

Figure 4: An oblique view of the lumbar spine, showing the "Scottie Dog." The pars is represented by the dog's collar, shown in faint red here. (Case courtesy of A.Prof Frank Gaillard, Radiopaedia.org, rID: 7552)

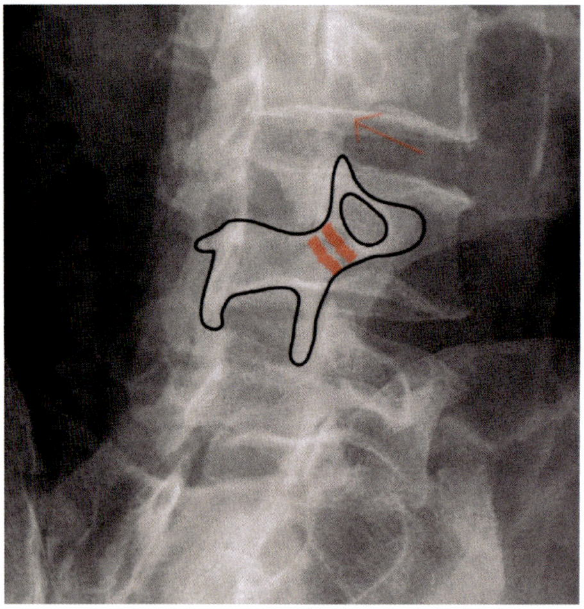

In spondylolisthesis, there is relative anterior displacement of the superior articular process, allowing the entire body to slip forward (Figure 5).

Figure 5: At left is a lateral x-ray showing an anterolisthesis at the L5-S1 level. In the annotation at right, the sacrum is outlined in yellow and the lumbar vertebral bodies in purple. The faint red lines outline the correct anatomic position from which the lumbar bodies have slipped. (Modified from https://en.wikipedia.org/wiki/Spondylolisthesis#/media/File:SpondylolisthesisL5S1.jpg)

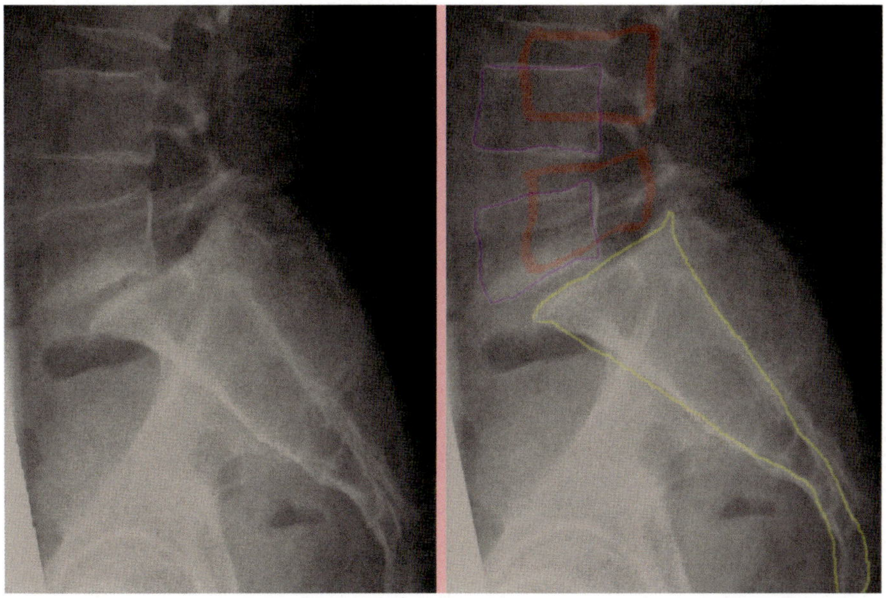

Spondylolisthesis can be graded based on magnitude of vertebral displacement. The superior endplate of the caudal vertebra is divided into quarters. The grade is dependent on location of the poster-inferior corner of the vertebra above. Grade 1 represents a 0-25% displacement, grade 2: 25-50%, grade 3: 50-75%, and grade 4: > 75%. Grades 1 and 2 are considered 'low grade' and grades 3 and 4 are considered 'high grade'. This distinction is important when developing an appropriate treatment strategy.

Advanced imaging may also play a role in the assessment of spondylolysis and spondylolisthesis in select circumstances. CT scan is the best modality for revealing the specific anatomy of the underlying lesion in spondylolysis, and thus can be helpful for delineating subtle defects. In patients with neurologic complaints or deficits on examination, MRI is warranted to further assess for neural element impingement. Bone scan (SPECT) is also highly sensitive for spondylolysis, and may be utilized in patients with a high suspicion for a pars defect with normal or inconclusive radiographs in whom cross-sectional imaging is undesirable.

EPIDEMIOLOGY

While the precise etiology of spondylolysis remains unknown, the pars defects typically occur in childhood or adolescence as an acquired phenomenon, as true congenital spondylolysis is exceedingly rare. This anatomic variant is present in 5 to 7 percent of the entire population, but can occur in as many as 45 percent of pediatric athletes involved in high risk sports. (High risk activities include gymnastics, Olympic weightlifting, football, dancing, figure skating, and wrestling.) This is currently the most common identifiable source of low back pain in adolescents.

Progression of spondylolysis to spondylolisthesis is uncommon, occurring in less than 15 percent of patients. Certain anatomic risk factors can help predict which patients are at increased risk of progressive listhesis.

L5-S1 is the most commonly affected spinal segment in isthmic spondylolisthesis (90%), followed by L4-L5 (10%).

Degenerative spondylolisthesis occurs in older adults. In the majority of cases, this occurs after the age of 40, though risk increases upon increasing age.

Isthmic spondylolisthesis is slightly more common in males, while degenerative spondylolisthesis is significantly more common in females (about eight times more prevalent) and occurs in approximately 10% of all women.

DIFFERENTIAL DIAGNOSIS

In the patient with unknown spondylolysis or spondylolisthesis presenting with low back pain, the differential diagnosis is broad. In the pediatric patient, this includes lumbar disc related pathology, lumbar muscle strain, Scheuermann's kyphosis, scoliosis, sacroiliac joint dysfunction, tumors (including especially osteoid osteoma), or infection (vertebral osteomyelitis or discitis). In the older patient, the differential diagnosis is similar but also includes degenerative disc disease or spinal stenosis without spondylolisthesis.

In a patient with confirmed spondylolisthesis, the differential diagnosis revolves around the specific etiology, and includes the six different types: dysplastic, isthmic, degenerative, traumatic, pathologic, and iatrogenic.

RED FLAGS

Pain that fails to relieve predictably with rest ("night pain") and associated constitutional symptoms (fever, chills, unintended weight loss) are always red flags for further investigation to avoid delays in making important diagnoses, such as malignancy or infection.

Signs or symptoms of cauda equina syndrome, which is a surgical emergency, include bowel or bladder incontinence, saddle anesthesia, and progressive lower extremity weakness. (Note that cauda equina compression from a high-grade listhesis requires translation of the posterior elements and laminae along with the body. Accordingly, compressions is highly unlikely in the setting of true isthmic spondylolisthesis.

TREATMENT OPTIONS AND OUTCOMES

The primary goal of treatment of spondylolysis is resolution of symptoms and return to activity. Radiographic healing of the pars defect may or may not correlate with the resolution of symptoms and is of secondary importance in the setting of isolated spondylolysis or low-grade spondylolisthesis.

There are three general categories of management strategy for patients with spondylolysis and spondylolisthesis: symptomatic treatment with analgesics and observation without activity modification/limitation (benign neglect); activity modification/limitation with or without bracing; and surgical intervention.

Benign neglect is most appropriate for asymptomatic or minimally symptomatic patients with isolated spondylolysis or low-grade spondylolistheses.

Activity modification is generally indicated for patients with spondylolysis or low-grade spondylolisthesis who are symptomatic. This strategy encompasses use of NSAIDs for pain control and physical therapy with a focus on stretching, lumbar spine flexion, core strengthening/stability as first-line.

For radicular pain that fails to improve with time and NSAID use, steroid injections may be a useful alternative.

Lumbar spine bracing may also be beneficial, particularly in the case of a failed trial of physical therapy or in an acute pars stress reaction spondylolysis, for which bracing is superior to activity restriction alone.

Surgical management is the final line of therapy for spondylolysis and spondylolisthesis. Surgery is rarely required for isolated spondylolysis without spondylolisthesis. Broadly, the major indications for surgery include refractory radicular symptoms, a progressive neurologic deficit, high grade progressive spondylolisthesis, and intractable pain or disability despite exhaustive non-operative management.

The goal of surgery for spondylolisthesis is to stabilize the unstable segment. This can prevent slip progression and reduce back or leg pain. Direct repair of a pars fracture may be considered in the absence of listhesis and at levels L4 and above in an effort to preserve lumbar motion. In degenerative spondylolisthesis, surgical options also typically include decompression (to address neural impingement) with or without concurrent fusion.

In general, the prognosis of spondylolysis and spondylolisthesis is very favorable. For symptomatic patients who undergo non-operative or operative treatment, the vast majority experience total relief of their pain and regain full functionality.

For patients with symptomatic spondylolysis, the majority will improve with observation and non-operative management. Only 15% of patients with spondylolysis will go on to develop spondylolisthesis.

For spondylolisthesis, the outcome is dependent upon grade/severity and specific subtype. Since most cases of spondylolisthesis are low grade, the overall prognosis is good. In these mild cases, non-operative management is successful in about 80% of patients. With regard to risk for displacement progression, dysplastic portends the highest rate (over 30%), while the most common type (isthmic) progresses in less than 5% of cases.

Severe spondylolisthesis portends a slightly worse prognosis, but the prognosis is still favorable overall. There is a higher risk of neurologic damage secondary to nerve compression, in addition to the risks associated with surgery (below). There is also a higher likelihood of persistent low back pain and disability, though surgery is successful in 85-90% of cases.

Specific complications of surgery include mainly pseudoarthrosis, infection, dural tear, neurologic deficits, and instrumentation (ie, the surgical hardware) failure. The risk of complications is generally higher for patients with degenerative spondylolisthesis given their increased age and medical comorbidities.

Note that excessive avoidance of activity may also impose costs on patients including deconditioning, weight gain, osteoporosis, and psychologic distress. It may be possible, thus, to be excessively conservative in recommending treatment.

RISK FACTORS AND PREVENTION

The primary risk factor for spondylolysis and spondylolisthesis is frequent hyperextension of the lumbar spine. Participation in sports such as gymnastics and football (and others in which the spine is extended) is associated with a higher prevalence of defects in the pars interarticularis.

The best approach for preventing spondylolysis is to avoid repetitive hyperextension of the lumbar spine. In addition, maintaining core muscle strength, flexibility and good bone health are important.

KEY TERMS

Spondylolysis, spondylolisthesis, facet joint, pars articularis, 'Scottie dog', spinal fusion

SKILLS

Understand the similarities and differences in the pathophysiology underlying spondylolysis and spondylolisthesis. Recognize the different subtypes and severity grading system for spondylolisthesis. Understand the non-operative and operative treatment modalities and their efficacy in the treatment of spondylolysis and spondylolisthesis.

CHAPTER 4.

SCAPULOTHORACIC DISORDERS

DESCRIPTION

The scapulothoracic joint is the articulation between the scapula and the thorax. It is not a true joint, but rather the broad contact between the inner surface of the scapula and the rib cage. The scapula is able to slide relative to the rib cage to allow for elevation and depression, along with protraction/retraction, rotation and shoulder abduction. When the arm moves relative to the body, approximately two-thirds of this motion is at the glenohumeral joint and one-third at the scapulothoracic joint. Three relatively common conditions are seen at the scapulothoracic joint. In **scapular winging**, the serratus anterior or trapezius fail to stabilize the scapula. (The muscle weakness is in turn caused by dysfunction of the long thoracic or spinal accessory nerves, respectively.) **Snapping scapula syndrome** is characterized by a grating sensation, often from overuse and scapulothoracic bursitis. With so-called **scapulothoracic dyskinesis**, abnormal scapula motion disrupts the normal glenohumeral joint mechanics and leads to shoulder pain. It is also possible to have a traumatic disruption of the scapulothoracic joint with high energy trauma. This is known as a **scapulothoracic dissociation**.

STRUCTURE AND FUNCTION

The scapulothoracic joint is not a true synovial articulation, but rather is the broad contact between the scapula and the thorax. The only ligamentous connection of the scapula to the body is via the clavicle: the medial clavicle is attached to the sternum, whereas its lateral end is attached to the scapula at the acromion.

There are 17 muscles that connect the scapula to the arm and the torso. Scapula-to-arm muscles include the four muscles of the rotator cuff, the biceps, the triceps, the coracobrachialis, the deltoid and part of the latissimus dorsi. Scapula-to-torso muscles include the rhomboids, the serratus anterior, and the trapezius. The serratus anterior muscle originates from the ribs and inserts on the medial scapular border; the trapezius originates from the vertebrae and inserts along the scapular spine. Dysfunction of the scapula-to-torso muscles can produce abnormal scapulothoracic motion and thereby disrupt normal glenohumeral joint mechanics. This scapular abnormality can thus be the cause of shoulder pain.

The scapula is internally rotated about 30° in the coronal plane and is slightly tipped anteriorly in the sagittal plane.

The scapula is able to move in multiple directions. These motions include elevation (as in shrugging the shoulders) and depression, protraction (moving the scapula laterally and anteriorly along the chest wall) and retraction (moving the scapula medially), and rotation.

Figure 1: A) The 4 basic straight motions of the scapula: elevation (purple) depression (red) protraction (yellow) and retraction (green). B) Medial rotation of the scapula (right scapula rotates clockwise as seen from the rear, medial side up). C) Lateral rotation of the scapula (right scapula rotates counter-clockwise as seen from the rear, lateral side up). (modified from https://radiopaedia.org/cases/scapulothoracic-joint-movements?lang=us)

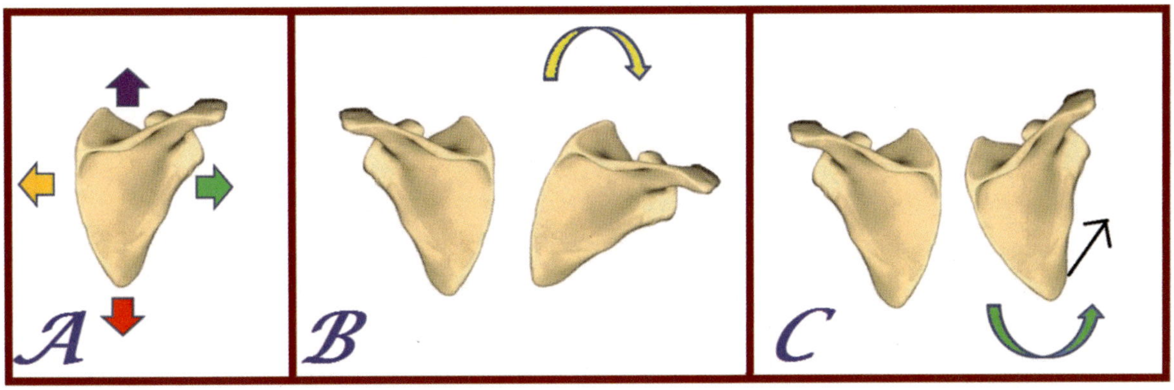

Motion of the scapula affects the position of the glenoid fossa, and in turn influences shoulder function. If the scapula does not move properly, the glenoid fossa will not be oriented for optimal contact with the humeral head. Also, about one-third of the arc of shoulder motion is at the scapulothoracic joint. As such, full range of motion of the shoulder requires normal scapular motion.

Motion of the scapula when motion is not desired can also lead to dysfunction; a lack of scapulothoracic stability can impede arm function as well.

The scapulothoracic bursae (plural) facilitate the gliding of the scapula on the chest wall.

Scapulothoracic bursitis is caused by poor scapular mechanics or a structural lesion (such as an osteochondroma of the scapula). Chronic inflammation leads to fibrosis, which can produce a snapping sensation. Snapping can also be the result of masses such as an osteochondroma or rib cage abnormalities (as may be seen with scoliosis).

PATIENT PRESENTATION

A patient with a scapulothoracic disorder may present with shoulder pain, especially with overhead activities, or with focal scapular complaints such as audible or palpable crepitus.

As always, a thorough physical examination is needed, starting with posture. Scoliosis or kyphosis that may contribute to bony incongruity should be noted. Active and passive glenohumeral motion should be evaluated, assessing scapular motion and the presence of crepitus, if any. Scapulothoracic crepitus is present in about of one-third of individuals without symptoms. Thus, this finding must be correlated to complaints.

Asking the patient to perform a "wall pushup" can reveal medial winging. The etiology of medial scapular winging is dysfunction of the serratus anterior or the long thoracic nerve that supplies it. There is weakness in protraction of the scapula, and thus the rhomboids and trapezius work unopposed.

Figure 2: Medial winging of the left scapula. (Courtesy of Khadilkar SV, et al. nn Indian Acad Neurol http://www.annalsofian.org/text.asp?2016/19/1/108/175435)

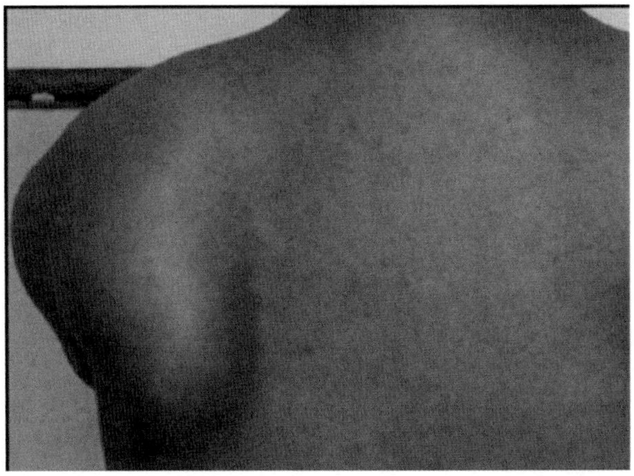

Lateral scapular winging is caused by dysfunction of the trapezius or the spinal accessory nerve that supplies it. In that setting, the serratus anterior works unopposed. This is usually an iatrogenic injury during neck surgery. The scapular flip sign can detect a spinal accessory nerve palsy. This sign is present when the medial scapular border "flips" or lifts from the thoracic wall during resisted shoulder external rotation with the arm at the side.

"Pseudo-winging" of the scapula can be seen without neuromuscular disease. One such instance would be when a tumor (e.g. osteochondroma) pushes the scapula off the posterior aspect of the chest wall. Psuedo-winging of the scapula can also be seen when patients learn to avoid painful positions by moving their scapula abnormally.

OBJECTIVE EVIDENCE

Plain x-rays will help detect osseous abnormalities. Snapping may be due to a mass. If a mass is seen on x-ray, then CT scans can be used for further definition. MRI may identify bursitis and soft-tissue masses.

Plain x-rays can also find abnormalities that upset normal scapular motion, including AC arthrosis, glenohumeral arthritis, thoracic kyphosis or scoliosis, and clavicular shortening (often due to fracture non-union or malunion).

Diagnostic injections of local anesthetic can identify or confirm symptomatic bursitis.

An EMG may confirm the presence of a nerve injury that is responsible for winging.

EPIDEMIOLOGY

Scapulothoracic disorders are thought to be rare, but may be under-diagnosed. That is, shoulder pain may be incorrectly attributed to primary disorders of the glenohumeral joint, when in fact scapulothoracic dysfunction is the true cause.

Scapulothoracic dyskinesis is usually found in athletes.

DIFFERENTIAL DIAGNOSIS

If snapping is present, the differential diagnosis is whether a mass is present or not. Imaging usually resolves this.

Scapular dyskinesis is often a diagnosis considered for a patient with shoulder pain that is not responding to treatment. Scapular dyskinesis is rarely the diagnosis considered first. Rather, it is a diagnosis made after all other diagnoses have been considered and rejected – a so-called "diagnosis of exclusion". It should be suspected in any patient with non-specific shoulder pain especially if the medial scapula is prominent at rest.

RED FLAGS

Winging is usually the product of nerve dysfunction, thus its presence should prompt a close examination to exclude any other neurological finding.

Two other points, not quite "red flags" but related to the general topic of vigilance, are worthy of notice. First, it is easy to miss a scapulothoracic diagnosis if the patient is insufficiently disrobed (or if the scapula is not palpated in lieu of direct visualization. As such, a shoulder examination with a fully clothed patient is a red flag for a possibly missed diagnosis. Second, the lung is near the scapula. Thus, if one is performing a bursal injection, it is critical to stay parallel to the undersurface of the scapula to avoid giving the patient a pneumothorax.

TREATMENT OPTIONS AND OUTCOMES

Non-surgical treatment could be utilized as the first line of treatment for patients with snapping scapula syndrome. Often, a non-surgical approach will alleviate patient's symptoms, especially patients with a problem with soft tissues. One to two cortisone injections can reduce symptoms associated with bursitis.

If there is a symptomatic mass, removal of the mass is indicated.

Arthroscopic bursectomy can be employed for patients who have a confirmed diagnosis (such as a positive response to a diagnostic injection and bursitis on MRI) who fail non-operative treatment.

The indications for surgery for those patients without an identified bursa or mass are less well defined. Resection of the superomedial or inferomedial angle of the scapula should be reserved for patients who localize their pain to precisely those areas and report adequate (albeit temporary) relief with an injection.

The mainstay of scapulothoracic dyskinesis is physical therapy, though if this condition is caused by a primary abnormality elsewhere, such as a clavicular or AC joint abnormality, physical therapy is unlikely to produce more than frustration. The underlying abnormality must be addressed.

For scapular conditions in general, physical therapy is focused on relative rest, increasing core muscle strength and balance, and improving posture.

Winging is usually monitored, though in some cases exploration of the nerve with neurolysis and possible repair is indicated. Winging that does not improve at all may require a muscle transfer or scapulothoracic fusion.

Snapping usually resolves over time. Snapping due to masses respond very well to resection. Because there can be a significant psychological overlay, surgery for snapping scapula in the absence of a mass lesion produces unpredictable and often disappointing results.

Scapulothoracic dyskinesis due to overuse also responds well to rest and rehabilitation. The outcomes in patients with scapulothoracic dyskinesis due to underlying abnormalities are governed by the response to treatment of those conditions.

Medial winging usually resolves over time as well, as it is caused by chronic compression. Lateral winging has a worse prognosis, as it usually caused by overt trauma to the nerves.

RISK FACTORS AND PREVENTION

Scapulothoracic dysfunction can be exacerbated by overuse. Recreational activities such as baseball pitching or occupations with repetitive overhead actions (e.g. carpentry) are also risk factors for this condition.

MISCELLANY

Scapulothoracic dyskinesis can be thought of as "SICK" scapula, which can remind the examiner of three associated findings: **S**capular malposition, **I**nferior medial border prominence, **C**oracoid pain and malposition, leading to dys**K**inesis of scapular movement.

KEY TERMS

Snapping scapula, scapular winging, scapulothoracic dyskinesis

SKILLS

Recognize scapular winging on examination.

CHAPTER 5.

DISORDERS OF THE ACROMIOCLAVICULAR JOINT

DESCRIPTION

The acromioclavicular (AC) joint is the junction between the clavicle and acromion process of the scapula. Subluxations and dislocations of this joint are colloquially called "shoulder separations" (perhaps to preserve the terms shoulder subluxation and shoulder dislocation for the glenohumeral joint). Patients with AC joint separations commonly present with pain after an athletic injury or fall onto the shoulder. Injuries to the joint rarely require surgical correction. They are generally managed non-operatively with excellent outcomes. The AC joint is also subject to early degenerative change. Arthritis of the acromioclavicular joint is a common cause of focal pain, especially in athletes.

STRUCTURE AND FUNCTION

The acromioclavicular joint is the articulation between the distal clavicle and the acromion process of the scapula (Figure 1).

Figure 1: An AP view of the shoulder, showing the acromion (Acr), clavicle and the AC joint. Also labeled are the humeral head (HH), the glenoid, the coracoid process (Cor) and the spine of the scapula (SS). (from https://radiopaedia.org/cases/normal-acromioclavicular-joint)

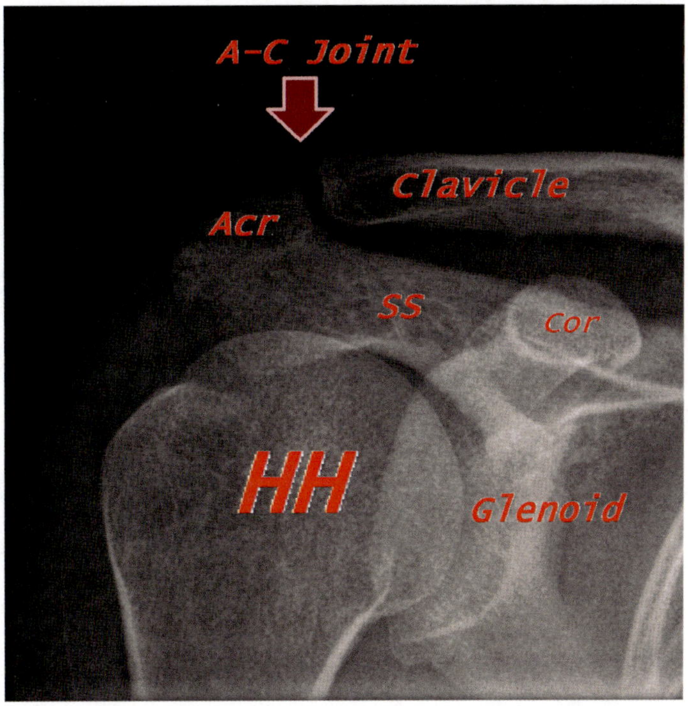

The joint is stabilized by the acromioclavicular ligament (also known as the "AC" ligament), which provides horizontal stability. The coracoclavicular ligament (also known as the "CC" ligament) provides vertical stability. The coracoclavicular ligament is actually a ligament complex composed of two parts: the more medial conoid ligament and the more lateral trapezoid ligament. The trapezoid is the more lateral, inserting about 3 cm from the end of the lateral (so-called "distal") clavicle, and the conoid inserts about 1.5 cm medial to that (Figure 2).

Figure 2: The ligaments of the shoulder: in gold, the coracoclavicular ligaments (trapezoid lateral, conoid medial); in purple, the coracoacromial ligament; in pink, the coracohumeral ligament; and in red, the acromioclavicular ligament. The glenohumeral ligaments are not shown. (modified from https://radiopaedia.org/cases/normal-acromioclavicular-joint)

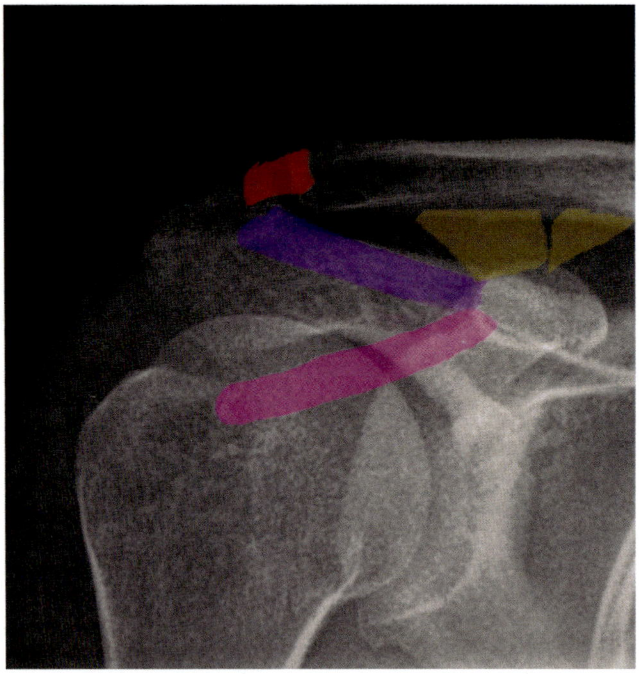

The coracoacromial ligament (also known as the "C-A" ligament), which runs from the coracoid process to the acromion, forms an arch that helps constrain the humeral head.

Some additional dynamic stability is provided by the deltoid and trapezius muscles.

The AC joint is neither fixed nor rigid, allowing for small amounts of gliding movement, typically accommodating about 5 mm of translation in every plane.

The joint itself is a synovial joint that is encased by a capsule that projects an intra-articular disc into the joint space.

If a person were to fall directly on the point of the shoulder, the acromion is forced inferiorly while the clavicle maintains its position. If the forces are greater than the tolerance of the ligaments, the joint will separate.

PATIENT PRESENTATION

Acute AC joint separations typically present after a fall on an adducted shoulder, often playing a contact sport such as football or hockey.

A patient will present with pain over the AC joint that limits shoulder range of motion, both passively and actively. Possible swelling or ecchymosis can occur over the AC joint with displacement of the arm and shoulder downward and forward causing the appearance of a prominent clavicle.

AC joint osteoarthritis presents with chronic discomfort localized to the joint. Patients may report difficulty using the arm or sleeping on the affected shoulder. At times there is a sense of clicking or snapping during use.

On physical examination, there is tenderness to palpation of the AC joint (Figure 3), a prominence of the distal clavicle (due to osteophytes) can be seen, and there is focal AC pain with cross body adduction of the arm (Figure 4).

Figure 3: Palpation of the AC joint.

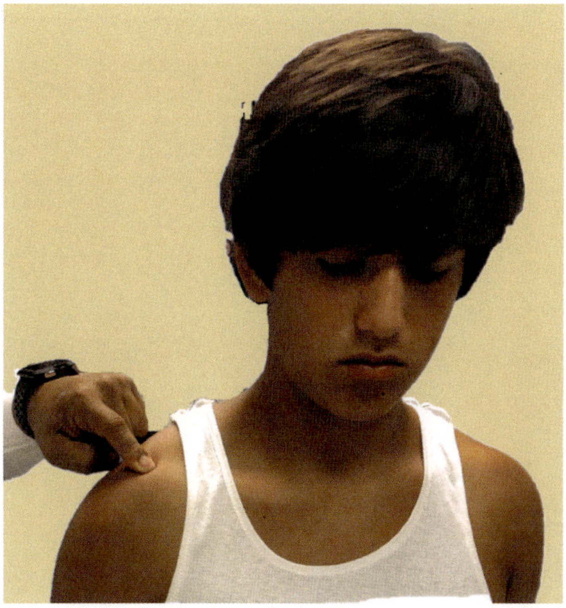

Figure 4: Cross body adduction of the arm is typically painful at the AC joint if that joint is arthritic.

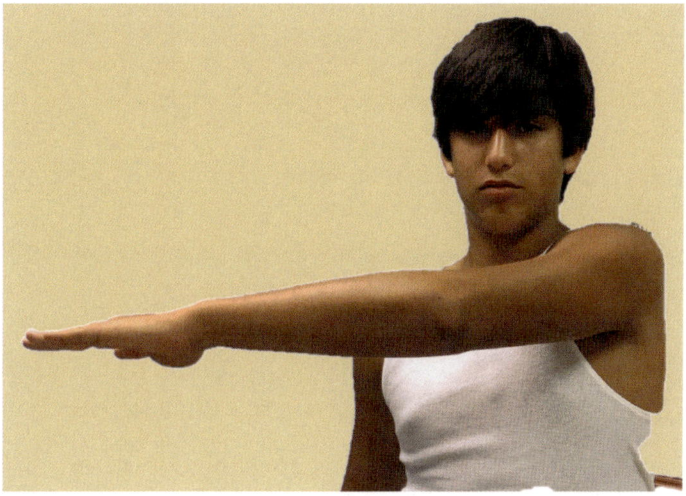

Often, AC joint osteoarthritis is seen in patient's who lift weights, particularly those that axially load the shoulder (i.e., bench press). In some of these patients, the pain can be rather acute, the joint may be swollen, and radiographs may demonstrate osteolysis of the end of the clavicle (regional osteopenia). This condition has been termed osteolysis of the distal clavicle, or more commonly, "weight lifter's shoulder."

OBJECTIVE EVIDENCE

AC joint separations are diagnosed by clinical examination and x-ray (Figure 5).

Figure 5: A downward force on the acromion (yellow) will tear the coracoclavicular ligaments (red). The distal clavicle will accordingly appear to be "high riding" but in fact the clavicle is close to normal in its position; it is the acromion that is lower than normal. (modified from https://www.ncbi.nlm.nih.gov/books/NBK493188/figure/article-17117.image.f1/)

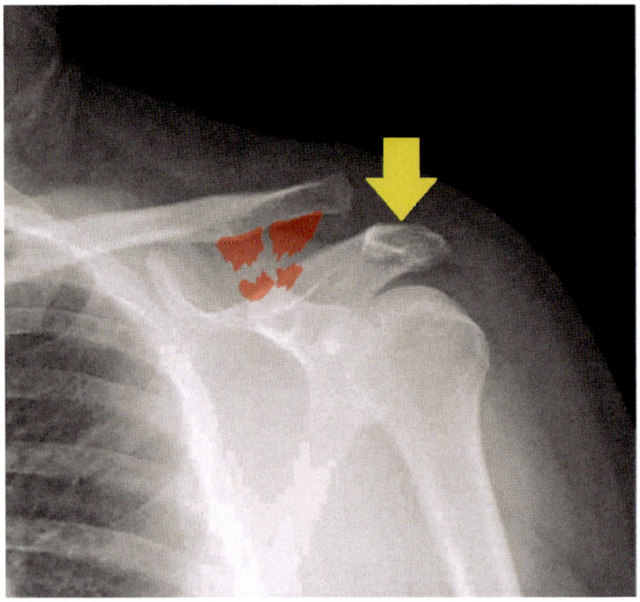

They are classified according to the amount and direction the physical separation seen between the acromion and the clavicle (Figure 6).

- Type I injuries are sprains or partial tears of the AC joint capsule without instability and have no visible deformity.
- Type II injuries include complete tears of the AC ligaments without involvement of the coracoclavicular ligaments. These injuries are characterized by slight displacement of the acromion from the clavicle.
- Type III injuries represent tears of both the AC and coracoclavicular ligaments and are associated with complete displacement of the joint.
- Type V injuries are basically Type III injuries with more marked displacement.
- (The rare Type IV injuries involve posterior displacement of the distal clavicle and Type VI injuries include inferior displacement of the distal clavicle underneath the coracoid process.)

It may be more useful to think of this classification as containing three broad categories: "nondisplaced"; "partially displaced"; and "displaced".

Figure 6: A schematic drawing showing three of the grades of AC separation. A grade I sprain has no displacement; a grade III has complete tears of the ligaments but only slight displacement; and a grade V has wide displacement. (See text for description of the even numbered grades). (modified from https://upload.wikimedia.org/wikipedia/commons/thumb/0/0f/ACJ_injuries_classification.svg/2000px-ACJ_injuries_classification.svg.png)

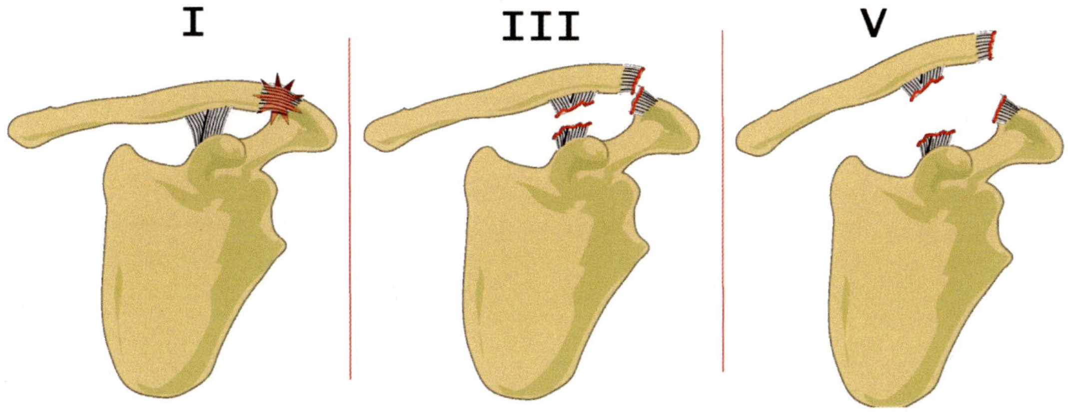

Radiographic assessment of the AC joint is best performed with bilateral anteroposterior (AP) views. This allows for side to side comparison of coracoidclavicle distance.

Axillary views can determine the amount of motion occurring in the sagittal plane, but these x-rays are also useful to make sure there is no glenohumeral joint disruption. In general, it is worth remembering that three views of the shoulder (AP, lateral and axillary) should always be obtained.

An AP x-ray with a 15-degree tilt cephalad (a so-called Zanca view) allows for a better visualization of the AC joint by removing the scapula from view.

AP radiographs while the patient is holding weight in each hand ("stress radiographs") can demonstrate an injury that is otherwise not apparent (especially separating a Type II injury from Type III injury), however this has the potential of causing further damage to an injured joint. Moreover, many physicians would offer the same treatment – non-operative management – independent of whether stress causes further displacement. This illustrates a key point: even a simple radiograph is a diagnostic test, and a diagnostic test should be obtained if and only if it will alter management.

In osteolysis of the distal clavicle, there may be widening of the AC joint due to complete loss of bone at the tip of the clavicle. The bone that remains may be tapered and osteopenic (faded, on x-ray) or have erosions and cysts. All of these findings reflect incomplete loss of bone.

Osteoarthritis can also be diagnosed with radiographs demonstrating joint space narrowing or growth of bone spurs.

EPIDEMIOLOGY

AC joint injuries represent about 10% of shoulder injuries in the general population, with nearly 50% of these injuries occurring in athletes. Nearly 90% of these injuries are low-grade and usually resolve within a week or two.

Osteoarthritis of the AC joint affects 5% of the adult population. Symptomatic arthritis of this joint is commonly seen in weightlifters.

DIFFERENTIAL DIAGNOSIS

A fracture of the distal clavicle can present similarly to AC joint separation, leaving the ligaments attached distally to the fracture site. Distal clavicle fractures can be ruled out with diagnostic x-rays although the two can occur simultaneously after major trauma.

It must be recalled that the physis (growth plate) of the distal clavicle is the last bone to fuse, and therefore up until age 25, a shoulder separation may actually be a growth plate fracture.

The very rare fracture of the base of the coracoid also presents with a superiorly displaced distal clavicle, but distance between the coracoid and the clavicle remains normal, about 10 mm, in most cases.

RED FLAGS

Although a majority of AC joint separation injuries are benign, the joint is not far from very important structures, including the subclavian vessels, brachial plexus and the lungs. High energy mechanisms of injury, especially with displacement, demand thorough scrutiny of physical examination and imaging studies to ensure that a pulmonary or neurovascular injury is not missed.

TREATMENT OPTIONS AND OUTCOMES

If the AC joint is not dislocated, non-operative treatment is recommended. Both Type I and II injuries can be managed with the use of a sling; the duration of course may be longer for an injury of greater severity.

Operative management is recommended for marked superior displacement, or any displacement posteriorly or inferiorly – that is Types IV, V and VI.

Operative management may be selected for some patients with complete but not exaggerated superior displacement, namely a Type III injury.

Surgery typically involves joint reduction, ligament repair or replacement with a graft, and reconstruction of the fascia that overlies the trapezius and deltoid muscles. Currently, sutures or combined suture and button constructs are utilized to hold the clavicle in place after acute injuries to allow for primary healing, or in chronic cases until a tendon graft has had ample time to heal. Historically, screws were used for this purpose; however, they have fallen out of favor due to hardware complications and worse outcomes (Figure 7).

Figure 7: An AC separation is shown at left. In the x-ray to the right, arrows point to the buttons used to anchor the suture holding the clavicle in the appropriate position during healing. (From Montoya et al. (2019) Surgical Treatment of High Degree AC-Joint Dislocations Using Double-Button Fixation Device. BAOJ Ortho 4: 025)

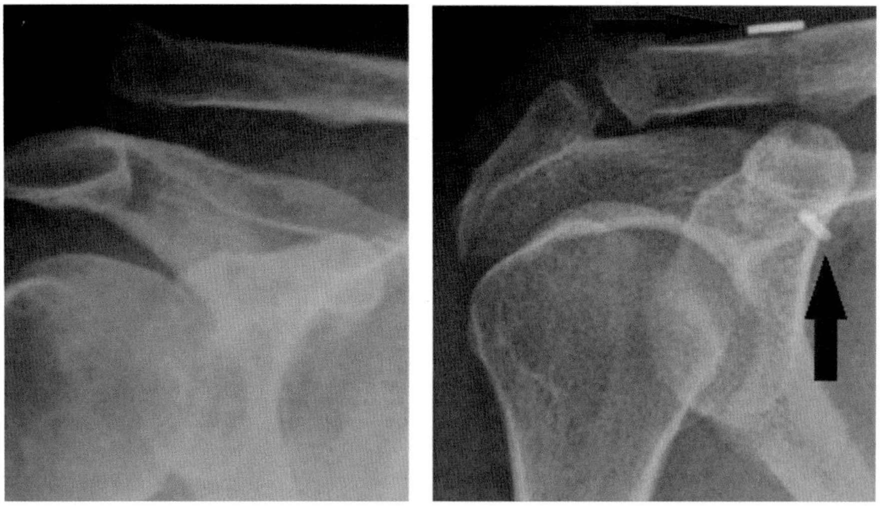

Post-operatively, patients typically use a sling for immobilization for six weeks. Active range of motion is initiated eight weeks after surgery, and resistance rehabilitation is started at the 12th week.

Treatment of osteoarthritis of the AC joint involves activity limitation and medication. Some may find temporary relief with injections of glucocorticoids into the joint space, however this relief is usually short-lived. In addition, it may be difficult to get a needle around the osteophytes (bone spurs).

A particularly symptomatic patient with arthritis of the acromioclavicular joint can be treated with resection, that is simply cutting out a small sliver of the distal clavicle and allowing a fibrocartilage scar to replace it.

The most common complication of AC joint separation is residual pain or limitations of mobility. This can affect 30% to 50% of patients.

Treatment of arthritis of the acromioclavicular joint with resection can provide good relief, as long as care is taken to not remove too much medial clavicle (which, by involving the ligaments, might produce instability).

RISK FACTORS AND PREVENTION

The single biggest risk factor for separation is in participation of contact sports (football, hockey, rugby).

Likewise, the risk factor for osteoarthritis of the AC joint is participation in activities that load the joint.

Neither of these categories of risk factors are particularly amenable to modification, though protective padding around the shoulders for football and ice hockey players (or for any sports that involves routine tackling and falling) has intuitive appeal.

MISCELLANY

Although the clavicle appears to be elevated in the case of an AC joint separation, what is seen, in fact, is acromial depression (due to the weight of the arm).

KEY TERMS

Acromioclavicular joint, coracoclavicular joint, synovial joint, Rockwood classification

SKILLS

Interpret classic history and physical exam findings to confirm diagnosis. Apply the classification of AC injury to formulate a treatment plan.

CHAPTER 6.

DISORDERS OF THE ROTATOR CUFF

DESCRIPTION

The rotator cuff comprises four muscles that originate on the scapula and insert on the humerus: the supraspinatus, infraspinatus, teres minor and subscapularis. Although these muscles have distinct effects on the humerus (often overlapping with non-rotator cuff muscles), the collective effect of the rotator cuff is to dynamically constrain the humeral head. Rotator cuff tears may be sudden and traumatic or gradual and attritional over time. Treatment ranges from benign neglect to surgical repair, depending on the functional loss of the injury and the patient's functional needs.

STRUCTURE AND FUNCTION

The rotator cuff is the collective term for the four muscles that originate on the scapula and insert on the humerus: the supraspinatus, infraspinatus, teres minor and subscapularis. Because their insertion is (somewhat) confluent, they are collectively designated a "cuff" (Figures 1 and 2).

Figure 1: Drawing of the rotator cuff muscles as seen from behind. (Modified from https://en.wikipedia.org/wiki/Rotator_cuff#/media/File:Shoulder_joint_back-en.svg)

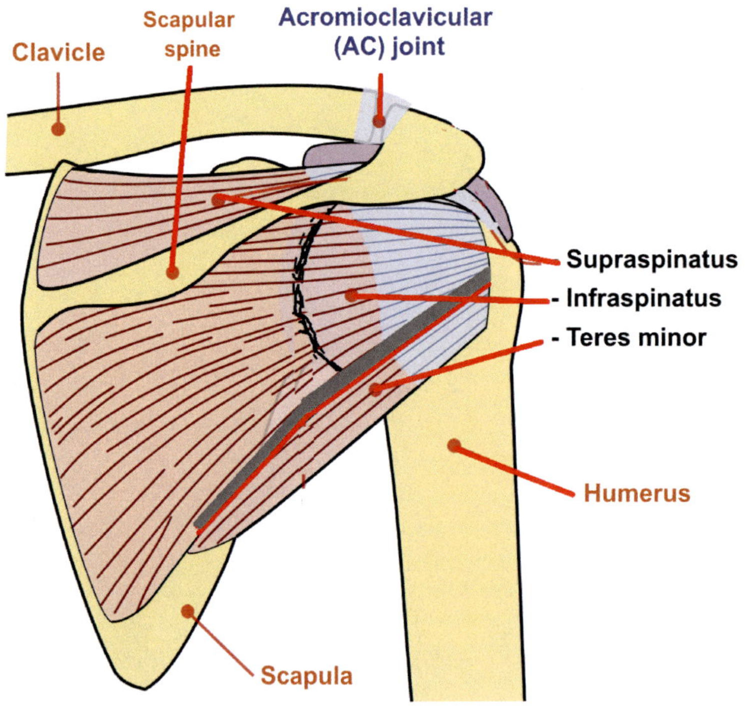

Figure 2: Drawing of the rotator cuff muscles as seen from the front. There are two lines pointing to the biceps (long head in blue, short head in red) and two lines pointing to the supraspinatus (tendon insertion in blue, muscle belly in red). Artistic license was taken to perform a small acromioplasty (removing the anterior edge of the acromion) to show the path of the supraspinatus tendon, which would ordinarily be covered by some bone. (Modified from https://en.wikipedia.org/wiki/Rotator_cuff#/media/File:Shoulder_joint_back-en.svg)

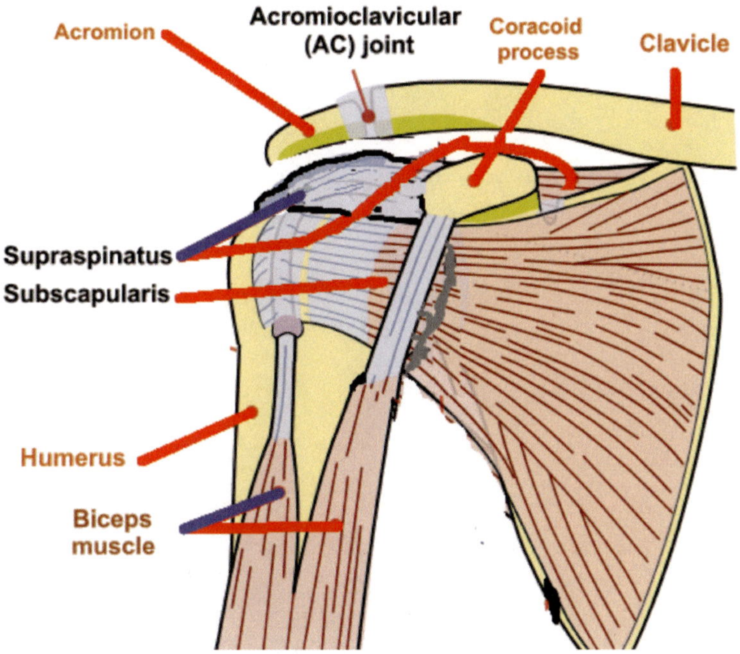

The supraspinatus originates in the supraspinatus fossa on the posterior scapula, crosses the superior humeral head, and inserts on the greater tuberosity.

The infraspinatus and teres minor originate in the infraspinatus fossa on the posterior scapula and insert on the greater tuberosity as well, posterior to the insertion point of the supraspinatus.

The subscapularis originates on the anterior aspect of the scapula and inserts on the lesser tuberosity.

The primary purpose of this cuff is to constrain the humeral head and initiate abduction and elevation. Recall that the glenoid is fairly shallow and that the shoulder is not a true ball and socket joint. If there was no constraint on the humeral head, the pull of the deltoid muscle, for example, will simply move the humeral head in a rostral direction. The rotator cuff primarily stabilizes the shoulder by compressing the humerus into the glenoid fossa. If the rotator cuff is able to constrain the humerus, a fulcrum is created, and the deltoid will then elevate or abduct the arm.

Additionally, the muscles of the rotator cuff can move the humerus: the supraspinatus produces abduction in the scapular plane; the infraspinatus and teres minor provide humeral external rotation; and the subscapularis produces internal rotation. Note that there is redundancy with other non-cuff muscles such that a rotator cuff tear – especially one developing chronically, over time – does not necessarily create a functional loss.

Complicating matters, it is possible to have overlapping diagnoses (some rotator cuff disorder coupled with some arthritis, for example), and it is possible to have anatomic abnormalities of the rotator cuff that are simply not responsible for the patient's symptoms – at least to the extent that fixing the anatomic abnormality may not make the patient better. This latter consideration is especially important given the recognition that highly sensitive testing modalities such as MRI are almost certain to detect abnormalities in people middle-aged and older, and it would be wrong to pounce upon an anatomic finding as a necessary explanation for a patient's pain.

PATIENT PRESENTATION

Patients with symptomatic rotator cuff disorders typically report pain in the anterior or lateral shoulder (greater tuberosity), especially with overhead activity.

There may be a prodrome of mild symptoms, with a superimposed worsening after an acute event.

On exam, patients might demonstrate weakness and pain with arm movement in the affected tendon's plane of motion. Because of the great redundancy of muscles coursing from the scapula or torso to the arm, some patients may have a so-called compensated rotator cuff tear, and have no functional loss despite losing the function of one or more rotator cuff tendons.

The physical examination should measure active and passive motion in elevation, abduction, and internal and external rotation. Specific maneuvers are shown in Figures 3 to 6.

Figure 3: Neer test. The patient's scapula is stabilized with one hand, while the arm is internally rotated and flexed to 180 degrees. If the patient experiences pain with flexion a lesion of the supraspinatus is suspected.

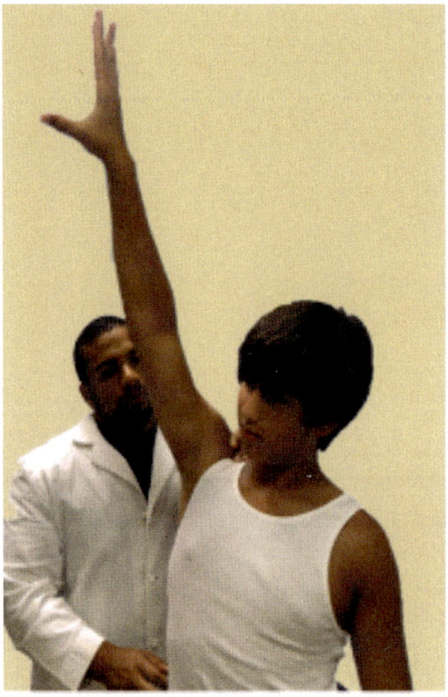

Figure 4: The supraspinatus test. The patient attempts, against resistance, to abduct the arms in the scapular plane (30 anterior to the body) with the elbows extended.

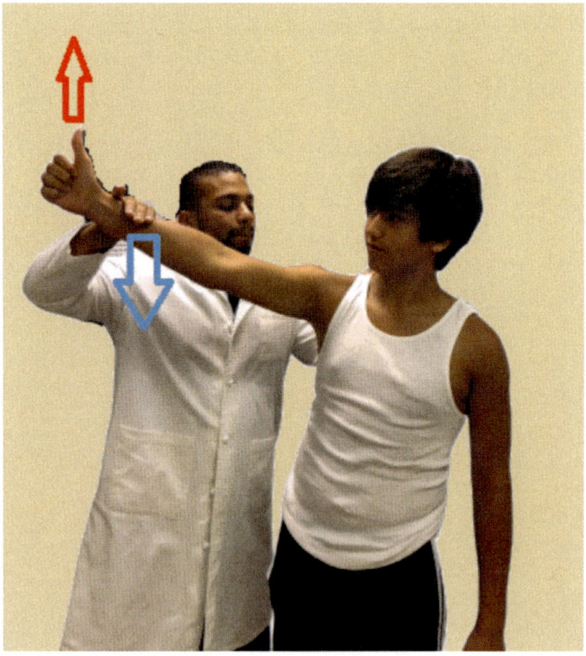

Figure 5: Infraspinatus/teres minor examination. The patient attempts to externally rotate the arms against resistance while the arms are at the sides and the elbows are flexed to 90 degrees. Holding the arms at the sides minimizes the effect of the deltoid.

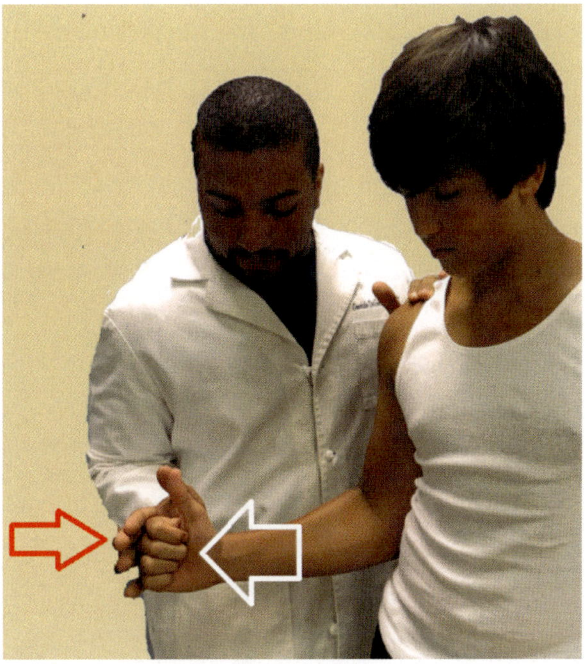

Figure 6: Lift-off test. The patient places the dorsum of the hand against mid-lumbar spine. The patient is asked to lift the hand away from the back. If the patient is unable to complete the task a lesion of the subscapularis is suspected.

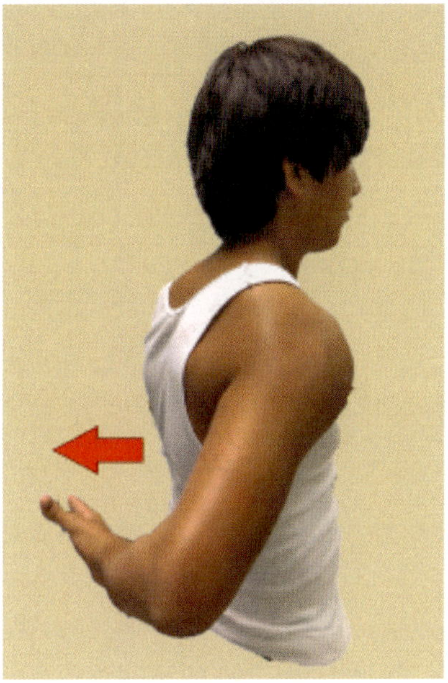

Loss of the bulk of the rotator cuff muscles on the posterior aspect of the scapula may suggest a chronic tear.

OBJECTIVE EVIDENCE

Plain radiographs are helpful in detecting arthrosis, calcific deposits in the tendons, and bone spurs. Large and long-standing cuff tears may also result in proximal humeral head migration relative to the glenoid.

Ultrasound is said to be both sensitive and specific for the identification of rotator cuff tears but is highly operator dependent.

Magnetic Residence Imaging (MRI) is also thought to be sensitive for the identification of rotator cuff tears (Figure 7). This modality is particularly useful for measuring the size of any tear, if present, and the presence or absence of tendon retraction, and muscle atrophy. The problem with MRI is that it may be too sensitive and can show things that are not necessarily clinically significant. In particular, MRI can detect a so-called partial thickness tear, in which the insertion of the muscle tendon unit is preserved however there is intrinsic damage to the tendon in its course. (The phrase "partial thickness tear" uses the word "tear" as it would be used in the phrase "wear and tear".) The relationship between this finding and the patient's symptoms is not assured.

Figure 7: An MRI of a torn supraspinatus. The edge of the tendons are shown in red. (Case courtesy of Dr Ahmed Abdrabou, Radiopaedia.org, rID: 36724)

EPIDEMIOLOGY

The majority of rotator cuff tears occur secondary to age related degenerative changes in rotator cuff tissue. As a general rule, a patient of X years of age will have an X% chance of having at least a partial rotator cuff tear on MRI, even if he or she has neither signs nor symptoms. Thus a "positive" test may not point to a meaningful diagnosis.

Rotator cuff tears in young adults are uncommon, but may occur following traumatic injuries, such as a fall on an outstretched arm.

DIFFERENTIAL DIAGNOSIS

Dysfunction of a rotator cuff muscle is usually indicative of a tear of that muscle-tendon unit, however a compressive neuropathy (of the suprascapular nerve) may mimic the functional loss of a complete rotator cuff tear.

The differential diagnosis for the symptoms overlapping with rotator cuff disorders includes subacromial bursitis, biceps tendonitis, labral disorders, adhesive capsulitis, glenohumeral or acromioclavicular arthritis, cervical radiculopathy, and shoulder instability.

Subacromial bursitis, also known as "impingement syndrome", is caused by inflammation of the bursa above rotator cuff tendons, mainly the supraspinatus. It can present with or without tendinopathy on MRI. This presentation was called "impingement" because it was thought to be caused by pressure from the acromion, though that is a misnomer: as noted politely in a leading journal, that theory has not withstood the test of time, based on studies that have shown similar outcomes independent of the presence of bony impingement on the cuff.

Rotator cuff dysfunction suggestive of a complete tear may be manifest even if the tendon is in continuity because of pain. This can be clarified by examination before and after an injection of an anesthetic (e.g., lidocaine) in the subacromial space. If after injection the patient no longer demonstrates weakness, preservation of the tendons' insertion can be inferred.

Bicep tendonitis may present as a rotator cuff disorder. (The long head of the bicep functions like a fifth rotator cuff tendon, one might say.) Bicep tendonitis can be differentiated on examination by producing pain with elbow motion against resistance.

Adhesive capsulitis (frozen shoulder) might present with signs and symptoms suggestive of rotator cuff disorder, but in this condition passive motion is limited as well.

Motion may also be limited with glenohumeral osteoarthritis. This condition is detected on imaging.

Cervical radiculopathy, especially involving the fifth cervical level, can cause shoulder or arm pain with muscle weakness. In this condition, however, there is usually also decreased sensation or paresthesias, and changes in symptoms with head and neck motion.

In young male athletes (especially weightlifters), the diagnosis of a pectoralis major (Figure 8) muscle or tendon tear should be considered. Pectoralis major tears typically occur during eccentric contractions, e.g., decelerating the bar in a bench press. Rupture can involve a tear of the muscle belly or tendon, or it can avulse off its insertion on the humerus. After the pectoralis major is ruptured, the patient will have limited horizontal adduction and internal rotation. Patients will demonstrate weakness with adduction and internal rotation, often with ecchymosis on the medial anterior aspect of the arm.

Figure 8: The pectoralis major has two "heads," named for their point of origin: the clavicular head which originates from the clavicle (shown in green) and a sternocostal head which originates from the sternum and rib cage (shown in blue). Both insert on the humerus and serve to adduct and flex the humerus. (https://en.wikipedia.org/wiki/Pectoralis_major#/media/File:Pectoralis_major.png)

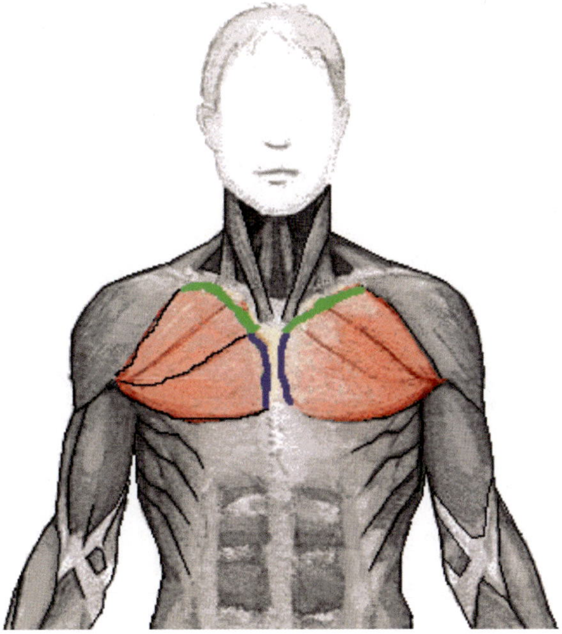

RED FLAGS

Neurological red flags include sensory deficits, winged scapula, or abnormal reflexes.

Left shoulder pain may have a cardiac origin.

TREATMENT OPTIONS AND OUTCOMES

Patients with rotator cuff disorders should be segregated into those who have had acute deterioration (notably, a sudden inability to elevate the arm) after trauma and those who are suffering from a more chronic pain-related condition. A patient who was highly functional, sustained an injury and had an abrupt loss of rotator cuff function is indicated for surgical repair– once imaging studies confirm the diagnosis, and that the remaining anatomy is amenable to repair. This repair should be performed expeditiously (within a month or so of injury), to prevent retraction of the tendon.

Tears of the pectoralis major should also be fixed, if possible.

Patients who have retained function but are limited by pain may do well with non-operative treatment. It is critical to avoid immobilization of the shoulder during recuperation as that will likely induce stiffness.

Physical therapy focuses on stretching of the posterior and anterior joint capsule, improving scapulohumeral coordination and strengthening the uninvolved rotator cuff. For example, if there is supraspinatus pathology, internal and external rotation exercises can be employed; the rationale of such a strengthening program is that a stronger infraspinatus and subscapularis may be adequate to contain the humeral head, allowing the supraspinatus to rest.

Subacromial injections may provide symptomatic relief. Because steroids are thought to weaken the tendon, by convention no more than a few of these injections are ever given.

Surgical repairs can be performed arthroscopically (Figure 9) or through an open procedure. The torn tendon is identified, debrided and anchored to the humerus (and if possible, sutured to the adjacent tendons as well).

Figure 9: At left, an arthroscopic view of a rotator cuff tear, denoted by the red star, no longer attached to the humeral head [HH]. The middle and right panels show a photo and drawing of the repair, respectively. (http://www.scielo.br/scielo.php?script=sci_arttext&pid=S0102-36162017000200164)

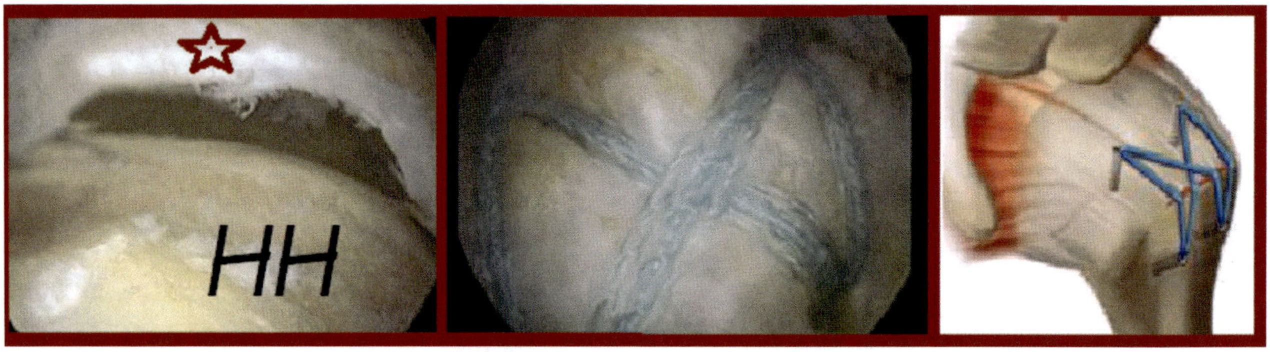

Most patients with rotator cuff disorders improve. It is not clear if this is necessarily from the intervention or the natural waxing and waning of the underlying disease.

Most patients who have surgery also do well, though interestingly outcomes after rotator cuff repair are somewhat independent of whether the tendon actually heals to bone: some patients do well even though the repair does not "take", whereas others with an intact tendon on postoperative imaging may have persistent symptoms.

(It is known that neglected tendon tears can lead to degenerative arthritis in the glenohumeral joint and that patients who immobilize their shoulders during painful flares can get stiff, bolstering our confidence that interventions are helpful, though it is certainly possible that some clinical improvement after treatment merely reflects the natural history of the disease.)

Patients with work-related injuries and those with ongoing litigation have poor outcomes.

RISK FACTORS AND PREVENTION

Risk factors for rotator cuff tears include increasing age, repetitive overhead activities and smoking. It has not been proven, but it makes intuitive sense to believe that maintaining the strength of all of the shoulder muscles will prevent dysfunction even if a given muscle were to degenerate or tear.

MISCELLANY

Mnemonic: The rotator cuff "sits" on the proximal humerus, and thus the names of the four muscles can be remembered by the four letters S I T S. The order of the tendon insertions also follows this mnemonic, coursing around the humeral head starting with the supraspinatus at the 12 o'clock position.

KEY TERMS

Rotator cuff, degeneration, tears, impingement, tendon repair

SKILLS

Complete upper extremity musculoskeletal exam and specific shoulder special tests. Interpret radiographs and MRIs for osseous lesions and soft tissue pathology. Demonstrate rotator cuff strengthening exercises to patients.

CHAPTER 7.

ADHESIVE CAPSULITIS

DESCRIPTION

Adhesive capsulitis, also known as frozen shoulder, is a condition in which inflammation within the capsule of the glenohumeral joint leads to its contracture and, with that, significant loss of motion and pain. Primary adhesive capsulitis describes the idiopathic presentation of these symptoms, while secondary adhesive capsulitis appears because of trauma, infection or other medical conditions such as diabetes or hypothyroidism. The painful phase of adhesive capsulitis usually resolves after a period of months, though some residual loss of motion remains even after the pain abates. Histologically, adhesive capsulitis is characterized by fibroblastic proliferation of the coracohumeral ligament and rotator interval, though very few cases progress to the point that a biopsy would be performed. Thus, adhesive capsulitis is usually a diagnosis of exclusion: it is the diagnosis applied to shoulder pain and lost motion where no other cause can be found.

STRUCTURE AND FUNCTION

The glenohumeral joint of the shoulder is a ball and socket joint in which the glenoid cavity of the scapula forms a socket for the humeral head. Unlike the femoral head of hip, the humeral head in the shoulder is not truly constrained within a socket: the glenoid is relatively shallow and thus the relationship of the humerus to the glenoid is akin to that of a golf ball on a tee (See Figure 1). This arrangement allows a far greater range of motion than is seen at the hip – with 120 degrees of unassisted flexion, the glenohumeral joint is the most mobile joint in the body. This motion, though, comes at the price of stability.

Figure 1: The "cup" of the hip and shoulder are outlined in red on these x-rays. As seen, the hip joint is considerably more constrained by the bony anatomy than the shoulder. When the shoulder capsule becomes more rigid and bone-like, shoulder motion becomes more like that of the hip joint.

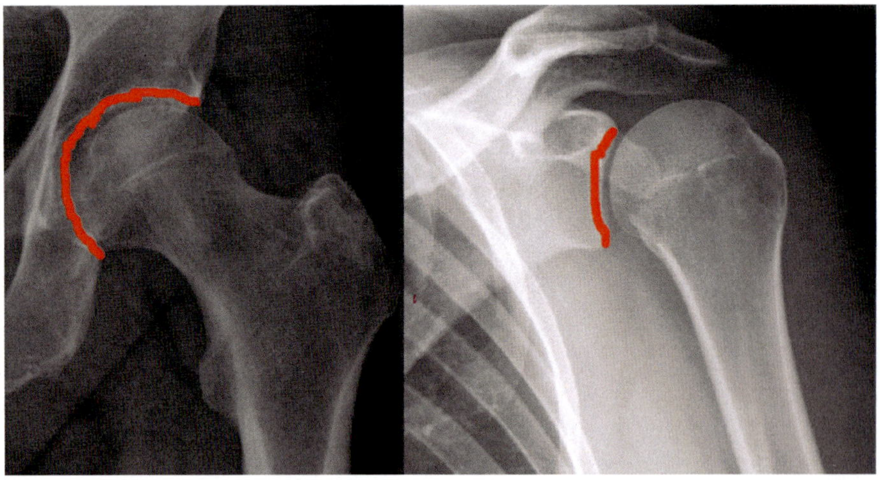

Stability of the glenohumeral joint is provided by the soft tissues. Dynamic (active) stability is a product of paired rotator cuff contraction, which tends to compress the humeral head into the glenoid cavity. The main source of static (passive) stability comes from the joint capsule (Figure 2) and ligaments, with some static stability coming from the glenoid labrum, which effectively deepens the glenoid.

Figure 2: The capsule, outlined in blue, holds the humeral head against the glenoid, substantially augmenting the (meager) stability offered by the bony anatomy. (Modified from Gray's Anatomy, Plate 327 https://commons.wikimedia.org/w/index.php?curid=108237)

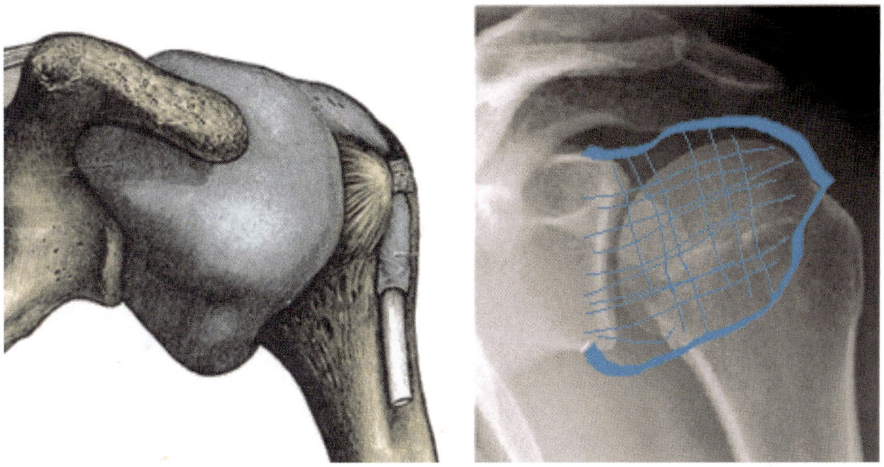

Adhesive capsulitis is caused by contracture of the capsule and intra-articular adhesions which physically tether the joint capsule to surrounding bone and tissues and further limit motion.

Histologically, early adhesive capsulitis is dominated by inflammation of the synovium. With disease progression, the inflamed synovium is replaced with diffuse fibrosis of the shoulder capsule.

Primary adhesive capsulitis is idiopathic. Adhesive capsulitis is also associated with medical conditions (such as diabetes mellitus, thyroid disease and stroke); medical interventions (such as prolonged immobilization, cardiac surgery and antiretroviral therapy for HIV); and injuries (such as rotator cuff tears or proximal humerus fractures). When there is an associated cause, the condition is designated as secondary adhesive capsulitis.

PATIENT PRESENTATION

The hallmarks of adhesive capsulitis are pain and decreased motion. Needless to say, there are many conditions which cause either pain or decreased motion or both; adhesive capsulitis can appear as an isolated condition or accompanying another shoulder condition.

Patients with adhesive capsulitis present with gradual unilateral shoulder pain that is often diffuse and worse at night. They also report an insidious onset of increasing stiffness. Some patients may "remember" a trivial trauma inciting the process, though this is likely a faulty attribution.

Clinically, isolated adhesive capsulitis has 3 distinct phases, namely: the painful phase, the stiff phase, and the resolution phases.

The Painful (or "freezing") Phase begins gradually, with no known precipitant. This phase, which lasts weeks to months, is characterized by diffuse, disabling pain that is worse at night.

The Stiff Phase is noted by marked stiffness that limits range of motion in multiple planes, interfering with activities of daily living. Pain is less intense at this point. This phase can last a year or longer.

Most patients enter a Resolution ("thawing") Phase during which motion improves, though often some limitations of range of motion compared to the contralateral shoulder remain.

On physical exam, patients with adhesive capsulitis have significantly reduced active and passive range of motion in two or more planes (see Figure 3 for normal ranges of motion). External rotation and abduction are the most commonly affected movements. Patients also have difficulty internally rotating. They might report problems scratching their back, for example, or hooking their bra from behind.

Figures 3: At left, the normal ranges of motion for forward elevation; in the center, internal rotation; and at right, and external rotation are shown.

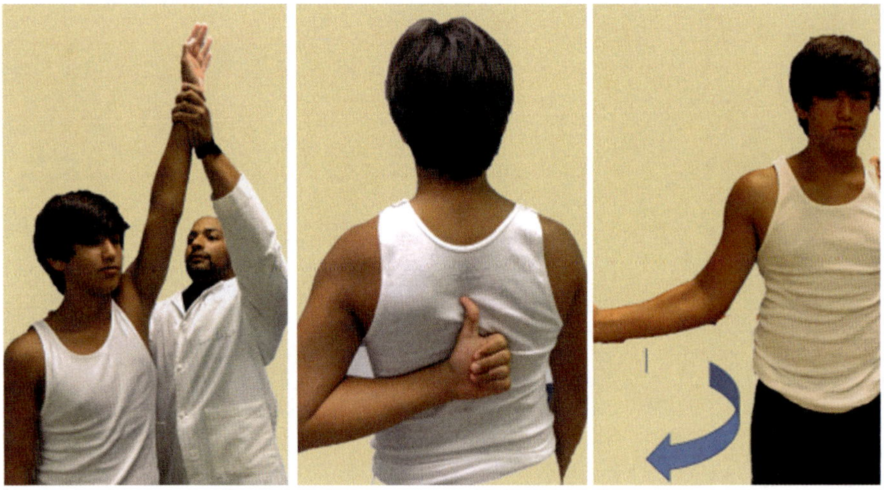

The critical finding of adhesive capsulitis is a loss of the end range of passive shoulder motion that is not limited by either pain or an intra-articular blockage. Adhesive capsulitis is a clinical diagnosis, made once radiographic evidence of underlying rotator cuff pathology and osteoarthritis is excluded. An inconsistent range of lost motion on examination precludes making the diagnosis of adhesive capsulitis. Lost motion of an inconsistent degree is more likely due to pain, malingering or other forms of active limitation, and not capsular contracture.

An intra-articular injection of an anesthetic can help eliminate the restrictions of motion imposed by pain.

OBJECTIVE EVIDENCE

Radiologic imaging does not diagnose adhesive capsulitis, but clinicians will often obtain plain radiographs to asses for glenohumeral arthritis or other shoulder pathologies. Plain radiography is usually normal in adhesive capsulitis.

Arthrography, in which the contracted joint is injected with contrast prior to imaging, can reliably diagnose capsular contracture: the normal shoulder accepts 20 ml of fluid without difficulty, but with adhesive capsulitis the shoulder usually holds less than 10 ml (Figure 4). Nonetheless, the degree of lost volume does not correlate perfectly with the degree of lost motion.

Figure 4: An arthrogram showing a reduced volume of contrast material within the shoulder joint. The red line outlines the border of the normal border of the capsule. (Modified from Radiopaedia.org, https://radiopaedia.org/cases/7545 ">rID: 7545</a)

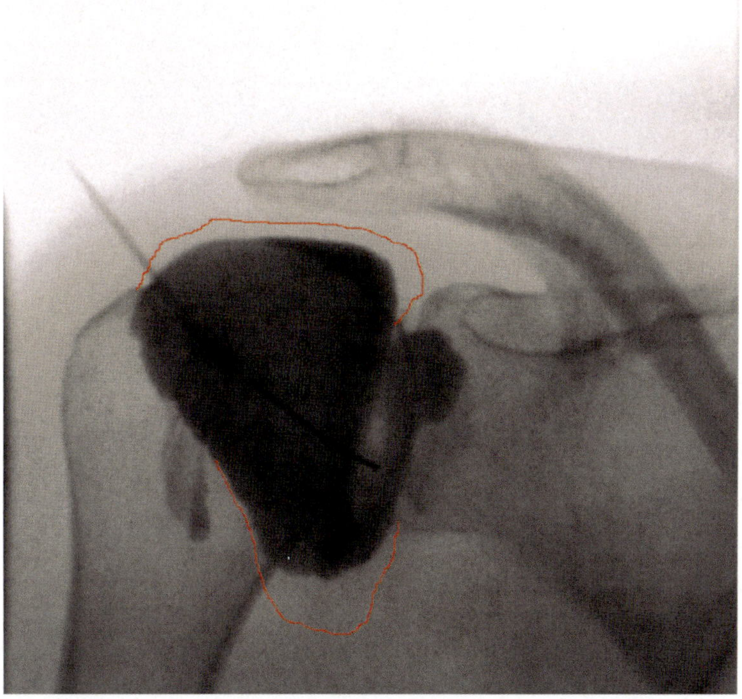

In primary adhesive capsulitis, there are no specific laboratory findings. Nonetheless, lab tests are commonly obtained once the diagnosis is made, to help identify a cause (e.g., diabetes).

Ultrasound can be used to rule out rotator cuff or bursal pathology. On ultrasound, thickening of the coracohumeral ligament and increased vascularity around the intraarticular portion of the biceps tendon may be seen with adhesive capsulitis.

Magnetic Resonance Imaging is also used to investigate the painful shoulder, as it is very sensitive for rotator cuff disease. MRI findings in adhesive capsulitis include thickening of the coracohumeral ligament and joint capsule with associated edema at the rotator cuff interval. MRI may demonstrate capsular thickening and decreased axillary pouch filling (Figure 5).

Figure 5: An MRI showing decreased volume of the axillary recess highlighted by the arrow. (Modified from https://radiopaedia.org/cases/adhesive-capsulitis-shoulder-3)

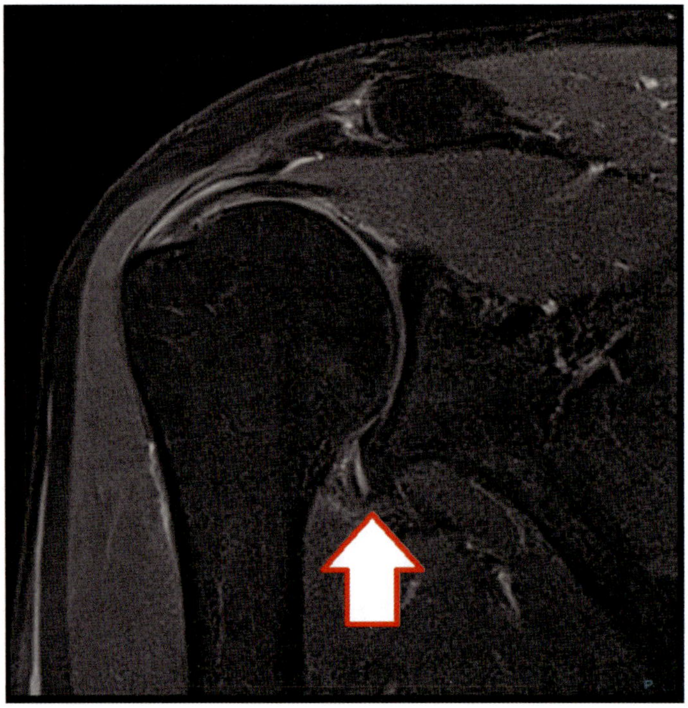

EPIDEMIOLOGY

It is estimated that approximately 5% of the general population, and 20% of patients with diabetes, will develop adhesive capsulitis in their lifetime. Adhesive capsulitis typically affects patients in their fifth or sixth decade, with a predilection for women. The non-dominant side is more frequently affected, though this bias may be a function of the patient's ability to not use the non-dominant side, which thereby allows the soft tissues to stiffen. Symptoms will develop in the contralateral shoulder in approximately 20% of cases.

DIFFERENTIAL DIAGNOSIS

The initial painful phase of adhesive capsulitis can overlap with subacromial bursitis/rotator cuff tendinopathy. Isolated adhesive capsulitis is usually not associated with repetitive motion or specific overhead activities. Also, adhesive capsulitis on physical exam is characterized by stiffness in more than one plane of motion. Adhesive capsulitis causes lost passive motion, whereas in cuff disease the range of passive motion is normal (though painful).

Another aspect of the patient history that can be very helpful in differentiating between different pathologies is the patients age. Primary adhesive capsulitis is rare in patients younger than 40 or older than 70 years.

Lost motion can be caused by glenohumeral arthritis, and therefore the diagnosis of adhesive capsulitis is reserved for cases in which no significant degenerative joint disease is seen.

The pain of adhesive capsulitis is usually found at the endpoint of motion, as the capsule is stretched. Until that is encountered, symptoms are minimal.

Sudden loss of motion may be caused by an unrecognized dislocation.

Other notable diagnoses to consider are neck pathology, cervical spine degeneration, diaphragmatic irritation, myocardial ischemia especially in an elderly female, or apical lung malignancy.

RED FLAGS

Night pain that awakens the patient from sleep may be due to occult malignancy that requires accurate diagnosis to guide treatment. Chronic shoulder pain with radiculopathy may suggest cervical spine pathology.

TREATMENT OPTIONS AND OUTCOMES

Adhesive capsulitis is a self-limiting disease, yet benign neglect is usually poorly tolerated. Due to the protracted course of adhesive capsulitis, which can take 2 years to resolve, many patients are unsatisfied with this lengthy period of pain and disability and are not comforted by the knowledge that the condition will eventually resolve. The pressure to "do something" is great.

The most commonly employed treatment for adhesive capsulitis is physical therapy to prevent soft-tissue contracture as well as to improve shoulder motion. This treatment may be limited to passive motion, as the patient is too symptomatic to do more actively.

Pharmacologic intervention is often included as empiric treatment in conjunction with therapy. Oral non-steroidal anti-inflammatory drugs may be given to modulate shoulder pain (whether they decrease capsule inflammation is not known).

Patients may also receive intra-articular corticosteroid injections for pain relief. The benefits of oral corticosteroids have not been shown to outweigh their risks. Intra-articular steroid injections may better optimize local concentrations of medicine and avoid systemic effects. Adding a large volume of saline may help lyse adhesions and stretch the capsule (a procedure known as "infiltration brisement" or "hydro-dilution"). This has a risk of capsular rupture, however.

Manipulation under anesthesia is generally regarded as a second-line treatment, chosen when non-operative treatments fail. Some potential risks include iatrogenic humeral dislocation or fracture, and soft tissue injury such as rotator cuff or labral tears.

Arthroscopic capsular release may be chosen in severe cases. Arthroscopic treatment has several advantages including visualization and exclusion of other diagnoses and focal lysis of adhesions in the coracohumeral ligament, rotator interval and inferior pouch (unlike manipulation, which stretches everything indiscriminately). Additionally, active range of motion can be performed soon after surgery to prevent new scar formation. Despite its advantages, arthroscopic capsular release is not without risks. Entering the joint capsule can be difficult due to a thick capsule and reduced joint space making insertion of trocars difficult and potentially damaging to the articular cartilage if excess force is applied.

The capsular changes in adhesive capsulitis shares some similarities to the fibrous contractures seen in Dupuytren's disease. The 2016 Richard A. Brand Award winning paper reported promising results using collagenase, an enzyme used in the treatment of Dupuytren's, to treat adhesive capsulitis.

Although adhesive capsulitis is a self-limiting disease, some patients may continue to demonstrate either shoulder pain and/or stiffness at 7-year follow-up.

Despite widespread use of physical therapy for the treatment of adhesive capsulitis, little evidence supports its use: a Cochrane database review was unable to confirm its benefit as a treatment. Still, retrospective case series evidence has demonstrated 90% of patients treated with a multi-directional stretching program were satisfied with their clinical result and given the pressure to take some action, this approach seems justified even in the face of poor evidence.

Treatment with oral medication has no high-level evidence supporting its use for treatment of adhesive capsulitis. One study has demonstrated that a 4-week regimen of naproxen or indomethacin had similar success for lowering pain levels. Risks of NSAID use include GI distress.

RISK FACTORS AND PREVENTION

Secondary adhesive capsulitis is associated with medical conditions such as diabetes mellitus, thyroid disease and stroke; medical interventions such as prolonged immobilization, cardiac surgery and antiretroviral therapy for HIV; and injuries such as rotator cuff tears or proximal humerus fractures.

Prevention of adhesive capsulitis centers on maintaining motion after an event of diagnosis that is associated with secondary adhesive capsulitis. Early shoulder mobilization after surgery is especially helpful for the retention of motion.

MISCELLANY

EA Codman coined the name Frozen Shoulder in 1934

KEYWORDS

adhesive capsulitis, capsule

SKILLS

Recognize adhesive capsulitis and distinguish it clinically by history and physical exam from other common shoulder pathologies. Describe treatment options for the management of adhesive capsulitis along with their risks and benefits.

CHAPTER 8.

GLENOHUMERAL ARTHRITIS

DESCRIPTION

Glenohumeral arthritis is defined by shoulder pain and stiffness from damage to the articulation between the humeral head and the glenoid process of the scapula. This arthritis may be idiopathic (osteoarthritis), or from autoimmune synovial inflammation (rheumatoid arthritis). Other known causes include trauma (including microtrauma from altered biomechanics or rotator cuff tears), gout, osteonecrosis, neuropathy (Charcot Arthropathy) and infection.

STRUCTURE AND FUNCTION

The glenohumeral joint is a ball and socket joint made by the articulation of the humeral head in the glenoid fossa of the scapula.

With little bony constraint, the joint is the most mobile joint in the body and consequently, inherently unstable. The joint is stabilized by static and dynamic restraints. The static restraints consist of the three glenohumeral ligaments and the glenoid labrum. The dynamic restraints consist of the rotator cuff muscles, the rotator interval, and the tendon of the long head of the biceps.

The glenohumeral joint has three degrees of freedom and functions to perform the following movements at the glenohumeral articulation: flexion/extension; adduction/abduction; and internal and external rotation. Forward flexion is also known as "elevation", and adduction is also known as "cross body abduction" or "horizontal abduction" (See figures 1 -4).

Figure 1: Shoulder elevation. Patients should be able to elevate the arm such that it is parallel with the torso, i.e., about 180 degrees.

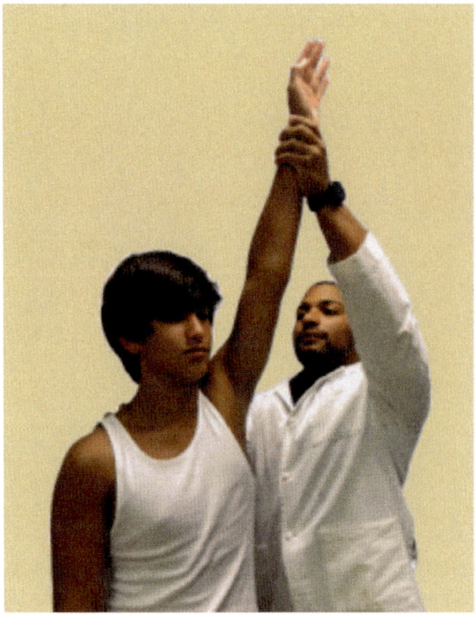

Figure 2: Shoulder adduction. Patients should able to reach across the midline, and ideally to be able to touch the contralateral shoulder.

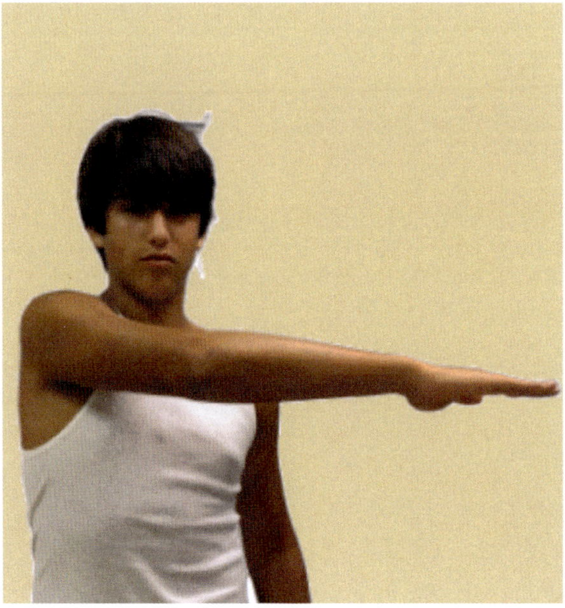

Figure 3: Shoulder internal rotation. Patients are asked to reach behind their backs. Internal rotation can be quantified by noting the approximate spinal level the patient can reach with his or her thumb, as shown.

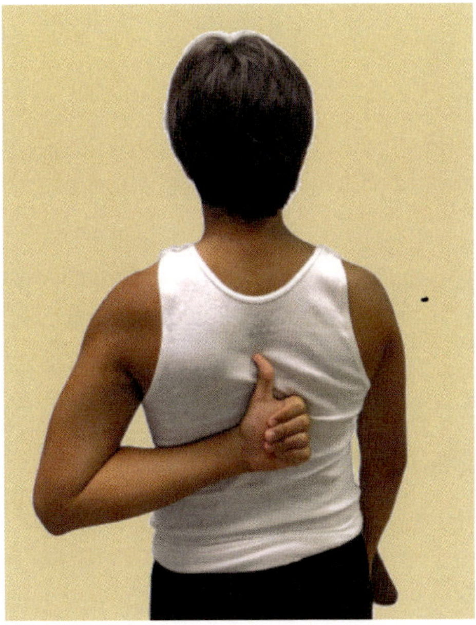

Figure 4: Shoulder external rotation is assessed by asking the patient to place his or her arm at the side, flex the elbow to 90 degrees and rotate externally. Because the scapula is not oriented perfectly with the torso, the glenohumeral joint is already externally rotated 30 degrees when the arm is pointing directly forward. The normal glenohumeral joint should be able to externally rotate an additional 60 degrees, as shown here.

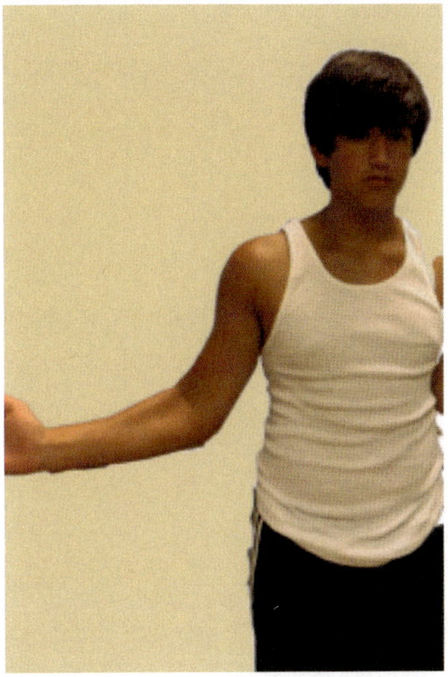

Glenoid version refers to the relationship between the glenoid cavity and the humeral head. It is a radiographic measurement determined by the angle between the glenoid line and the line perpendicular to the scapular axis. The glenoid is normally slightly retroverted. In addition, the humeral head and neck are also retroverted from the humeral shaft (with the anterior plane defined by the position of the humeral epicondyles at the elbow). Normal humeral version is 20-30° of retroversion. Deviations from normal version can disturb normal mechanics and lead to arthritic changes.

In glenohumeral arthritis, the articular cartilage of the humeral head or glenoid or both is damaged. As in the arthritis of many other joints, glenohumeral arthritis can affect the subchondral bone as well.

The most common etiology of glenohumeral arthritis is primary osteoarthritis (OA). OA is characterized by progressive degeneration of articular cartilage, dense subchondral bone growth, osteophyte formation, glenoid erosion, and displacement of the humeral head.

Additional Causes of Glenohumeral Arthritis

- *Rheumatoid Arthritis (RA)* – Systemic autoimmune disease of the synovium. Synovial inflammation and soft tissue break down at the shoulder results in wear of the glenoid articular cartilage and medialization of the humeral head.
- *Post-traumatic arthritis* – Disruption of the articular surface can occur after a humeral fracture or dislocation. The damage with dislocation can be from the impact of the dislocation episode or from microtrauma inflicted by chronic instability.
- *Crystalline arthritis* – Gout and Calcium Pyrophosphate Dihydrate Deposition Disease (CPPD) result in the deposition of crystals within the joint space which cause synovial inflammation and resultant cartilage damage.
- *Osteonecrosis* – Morphological and arthritic changes result from loss of blood supply to the humeral head. Osteonecrosis can appear from trauma, use/abuse of alcohol or steroids, hemoglobinopathies, among other causes. It may also be idiopathic (no known cause).
- *Charcot Arthropathy* – Loss of sensation and proprioception in the joint results in repetitive microtrauma and joint degeneration. Charcot Arthropathy of the shoulder is often related to cervical spine syrinx.
- *Rotator cuff arthropathy* – Tears of the rotator cuff tendons disturb normal biomechanics (as the rotator cuff is an important shoulder stabilizer). Such tears produce abnormal humeral head contact, leading to breaking down of the articular surfaces.
- *Septic Arthritis* – The white cell response to infection can damage articular cartilage.

PATIENT PRESENTATION

Patients with glenohumeral arthritis present with shoulder pain and stiffness. Taking a thorough history with these patients is key as it can determine the etiology of the disease.

The clinical presentation depends on the underlying cause of the arthritis.

Patients with glenohumeral osteoarthritis are typically over 50 years old and present with a chief complaint of pain. The pain is usually insidious in onset, progressive, chronic, and worsens with activity. Discomfort may lead to nocturnal awakening, especially when lying on the affected side, and patients typically have functional limitations due to a decreased range of motion. On physical exam, the affected extremity may be atrophic secondary to disuse. Patients have tenderness over the posterior joint line and crepitus with motion of the joint. The most dramatic finding is typically decreased range of motion which is most pronounced with external rotation.

Patients with rheumatoid arthritis present with pain, decreased range of motion, crepitation, and effusions in multiple joints. The effects typically evolve slowly and insidiously. The shoulder is rarely the first joint affected and it is almost never the only affected joint.

In cuff tear arthropathy, patients are usually significantly disabled and are unable to raise their affected arm. Inspection may show hollowing around the scapula secondary to cuff muscle atrophy.

A number of other disease processes, including osteonecrosis, recurrent glenohumeral dislocations, and posttraumatic articular incongruity can lead to destruction of the glenohumeral articular cartilage. In most cases, this results in secondary osteoarthritis and has symptoms similar to primary osteoarthritis although the history will suggest this secondary cause.

Of note, septic arthritis may hurt even without motion, but symptoms are worsened with activity.

OBJECTIVE EVIDENCE

Imaging of the glenohumeral joint starts with radiographs taken at three views: AP, lateral and scapular (also known as a "Y") view. Findings on these radiographs often lead to the etiology of the arthritis (Figure 5).

Figure 5: Osteoarthritis of the shoulder is shown, with bony sclerosis, osteophyte formation and superior migration of the humeral head. (Case courtesy of Radiopedia case 43425.)

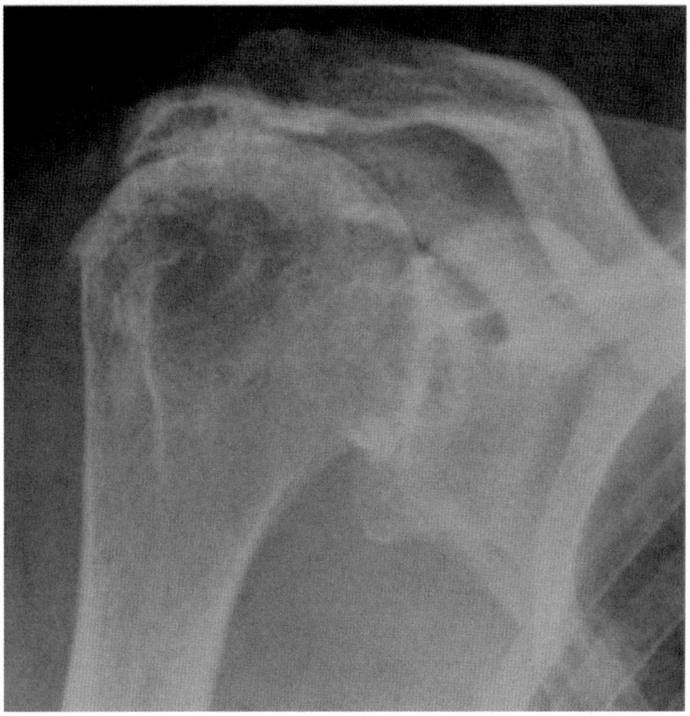

Advanced imaging such as CT and MRI are indicated for pre-operative planning as they provide the surgeon with enhanced imaging of glenoid morphology and rotator cuff pathology.

For the most part, no laboratory tests are necessary for the diagnosis of glenohumeral arthritis. However, if an inflammatory or crystalline arthropathy is suspected, specific labs may be indicated. Namely, ESR, CRP, Rheumatoid factor, and Anti-CCP antibodies for RA and synovial fluid analysis for crystalline arthropathies.

EPIDEMIOLOGY

Arthritis of the glenohumeral joint typically affects patients in the sixth decade of life and on. Of the large joints, the glenohumeral joint trails the hip and knee in the incidence of arthritis–perhaps because a person can avoid using his or her shoulder in a way not possible with the weight bearing joints. Yet because of this relative underuse potential, the true incidence of glenohumeral arthritis remains undetermined.

DIFFERENTIAL DIAGNOSIS

Shoulder pain with decreased mobility is a common presentation. After the clinician has determined the shoulder pain to be glenohumeral in origin, the following diagnoses, in the alternative, or in addition to arthritis should be considered:

- Rotator cuff impingement and tendinopathy,
- Rotator cuff tear,
- Adhesive capsulitis,
- Shoulder instability with or without bony or labral damage,
- Locked posterior dislocations in elderly patients.

Clinically, these injuries can appear identical to glenohumeral arthritis and radiographic studies are needed to determine the etiology of the shoulder pain.

Of note, rotator cuff tears have a 5-10% incidence with osteoarthritis of the glenohumeral joint and a 25-50% incidence with rheumatoid arthritis.

RED FLAGS

Arthritis of the glenohumeral joint is a chronic condition that rarely requires emergency treatment. However, a patient who presents with fever, chills, and fatigue in addition to pain, swelling, warmth, and erythema of the shoulder should be promptly evaluated for a septic shoulder. Exuberant arthritis limited to just the shoulder(s) should prompt a cervical examination for a syrinx.

Shoulder pain might be caused by lung cancers in the superior aspect of the lung (so-called Pancoast tumors). This should not be missed when reviewing the radiographs.

TREATMENT OPTIONS AND OUTCOMES

Mainstays of non-operative treatment for glenohumeral arthritis consist of physical therapy, NSAIDs, activity modification, and injections. NSAIDs reduce pain and inflammation, while physical therapy works to improve range of motion and strengthen the surrounding musculature.

RA can be very well controlled with disease-modifying antirheumatic drugs (DMARD). Intraarticular injections of corticosteroids act to reduce inflammation. However, arthritis is a progressive disease and medical treatment exhausts quickly.

End stage degenerative joint disease can be treated with joint replacement: Hemiarthroplasty; Total Shoulder Arthroplasty; and Reverse Shoulder Arthroplasty.

Hemiarthroplasty

A hemiarthroplasty involves replacing the humeral head with a stemmed prosthesis. It is indicated for patients who have failed non-operative treatment with an intact glenoid and articular damage to the humerus. The best results are seen in patients with concentric glenoids and intact rotator cuffs. This operation is technically easier than adding a glenoid replacement, but usually provides less symptomatic relief. Hemiarthroplasty is also used to treat fracture of the humeral head.

Total Shoulder Arthroplasty

In a total shoulder arthroplasty, the arthritic humeral head is replaced with a metal ball fixed to a stem inserted into the humeral shaft and the glenoid is resurfaced with a polyethylene insert (Figure 6). This procedure is best for patients with a moderate to low activity level. Patients need good bone stock and an intact or repairable rotator cuff. Patients treated with total shoulder arthroplasty see good pain relief and reliable range of motion with a 10-year survival rate of 92-95%. Common complications include component loosening, infection, fracture nerve injury, and rotator cuff tear.

Figure 6: Total shoulder arthroplasty. The glenoid component is made of plastic and not readily apparent on x-ray (unless you look for it); it is outlined in the reproduction at right. (courtesy https://www.ncbi.nlm.nih.gov/pmc/articles/PMC3093753/)

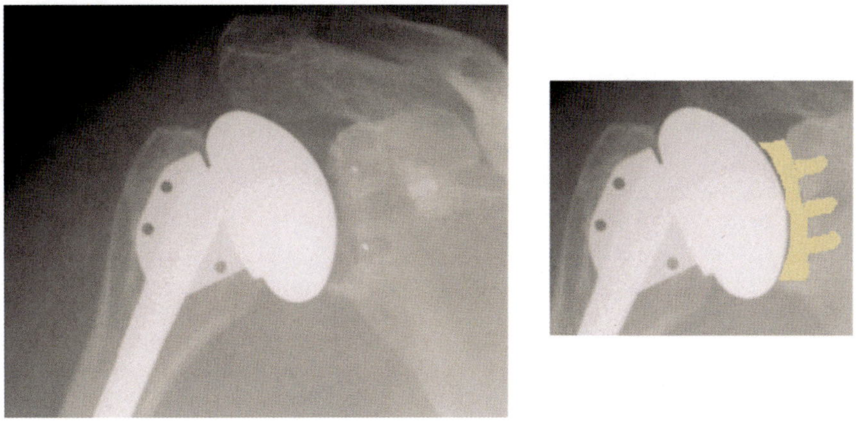

Reverse Shoulder Arthroplasty

In a reverse shoulder arthroplasty, the glenoid socket is replaced with a metal ball and secured to the scapula and the humeral head is replaced with a cup attached to a stem which functions as a socket (Figure 7). This is the opposite anatomic arrangement of the native glenohumeral joint. This arrangement provides stability in the absence of a functioning rotator cuff. It is indicated for rotator cuff arthropathy, severe proximal humerus fractures, failed total shoulder arthropathy, and glenohumeral deformities that cannot be reconstructed otherwise. This operation can dramatically increase the function of the shoulder and provide excellent pain relief.

Figure 7: A reverse shoulder arthroplasty.

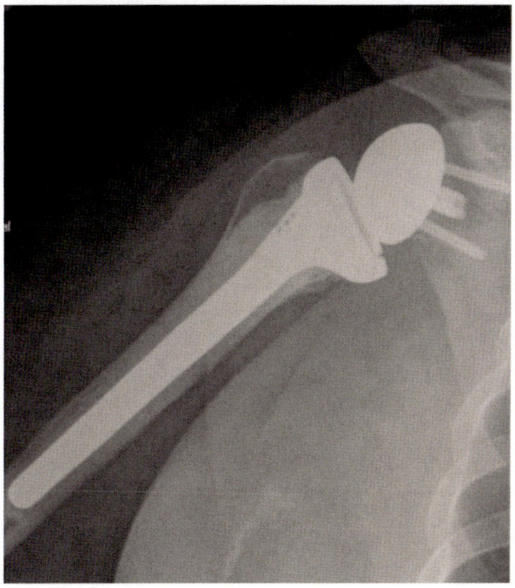

Shoulder Arthrodesis
An arthrodesis involves the surgical resection and fusion of the glenohumeral joint. This operation is indicated for laborers unwilling to alter their activities, uncontrolled joint sepsis, recurrent shoulder instability, loss of rotator cuff and deltoid musculature, brachial plexus plexopathies, and salvage for failed total shoulder arthroplasty. Because there is a lot of motion between the scapula and thorax, this operation is tolerated better than an analogous fusion of the hip joint. Nonetheless, most patients are happier with a joint replacement.

RISK FACTORS AND PREVENTION

Age is one of the primary risks for the development of glenohumeral arthritis. Females display higher incidences of both OA and RA. Glenohumeral arthritis is associated with activities that put high strain on the glenohumeral joint. However, many patients develop arthritis of the shoulder without a decipherable cause.

Lifting heavy weights, either at work or for recreation, increases the chances of developing glenohumeral osteoarthritis.

The incidence of glenohumeral arthritis increase with a history of trauma and prior surgery to the shoulder. Certain studies have shown that over 50% of patients with a primary anterior shoulder dislocation go on to develop some degree of glenohumeral arthritis at 25 years follow-up.

MISCELLANY

The characteristic osteophyte of glenohumeral arthritis is termed a goat's beard (Figure 8).

Figure 8: An inferior osteophyte suggestive of a goat's beard. (courtesy https://www.orthopaedicsone.com/display/MSKMed/Arthritis+of+the+Gleno-humeral+joint)

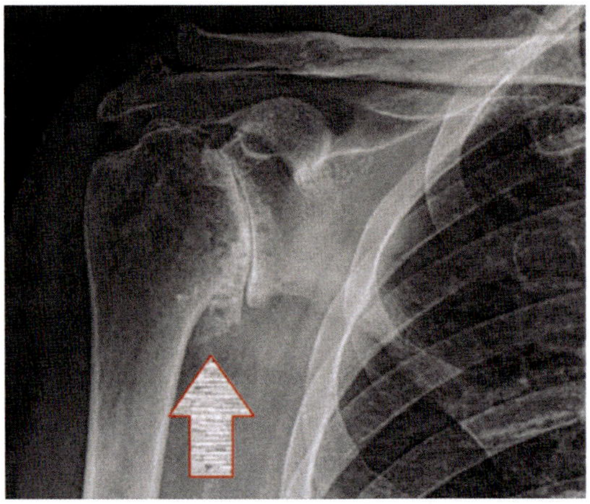

KEY TERMS

Glenohumeral arthritis, osteoarthritis, rheumatoid arthritis, articular cartilage, arthroplasty

SKILLS

Recognize and describe the deformities of the glenohumeral joint caused by arthritis. Recognize the potential etiologies of glenohumeral arthritis. Recognize the clinical and radiographic signs of glenohumeral arthritis. Describe the different treatment modalities for glenohumeral arthritis.

CHAPTER 9.

GLENOHUMERAL INSTABILITY

DESCRIPTION

Glenohumeral instability is defined as an inability to maintain the humeral head centered in the glenoid fossa. This problem is typically caused by either a traumatic rupture of the capsule and ligaments (usually following a complete dislocation or partial dislocation/subluxation), or by generalized laxity of the soft tissue. In the case of post-dislocation instability, the shoulder is unstable in only one plane (namely, in the direction of the dislocation), whereas with generalized laxity, the instability is multidirectional. Patients with glenohumeral instability may suffer repeat episodes of subluxation in which the joint surfaces are damaged. In very broad terms, instability from trauma is amenable to surgical repair, whereas multidirectional is not. Multidirectional instability is treated with physical therapy to strengthen the rotator cuff, but this does not always stabilize the joint sufficiently.

STRUCTURE AND FUNCTION

Unlike the femoroacetabular joint of the hip and humeroulnar joint at the elbow, the glenohumeral joint has little static stability provided by the bony anatomy. The humeral head is not constrained by the (relatively shallow) glenoid fossa; rather, only a small portion of the humeral head articulates with the glenoid (Figure 1).

Figure 1: A CT scan of the shoulder, showing the mismatch between the size of the glenoid (yellow) and the size of the humeral head (red). (https://radiopaedia.org/cases/normal-ct-shoulder-2)

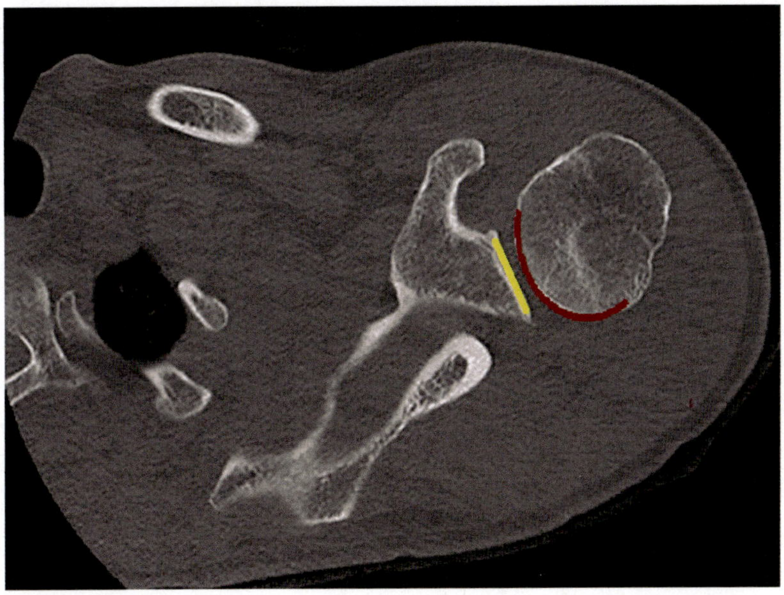

Accordingly, the shoulder relies on both dynamic (active) and static (passive) soft-tissue stabilizers. The main static stabilizers of the shoulder are the ligaments and capsular tissue. Some additional static stability is provided by the labrum, a lip of cartilage around the glenoid that deepens the socket.

There are regions of the capsule which are identified as distinct ligaments (Figure 2). The superior glenohumeral ligament provides stability with the arm at the side, the middle glenohumeral provides restraint with the arm partially abducted and the inferior glenohumeral ligament is the primary stabilizer with the arm fully abducted.

Figure 2: The ligaments connecting the humerus to the scapula. The coracohumeral ligament is shown in faint black; the capsule is outlined in red. The capsule itself comprises the superior (green) middle (pink) and inferior (yellow) glenohumeral ligaments. (Annotations on x-ray courtesy of https://radiopaedia.org/cases/external-and-internal-rotation-views-of-the-shoulder)

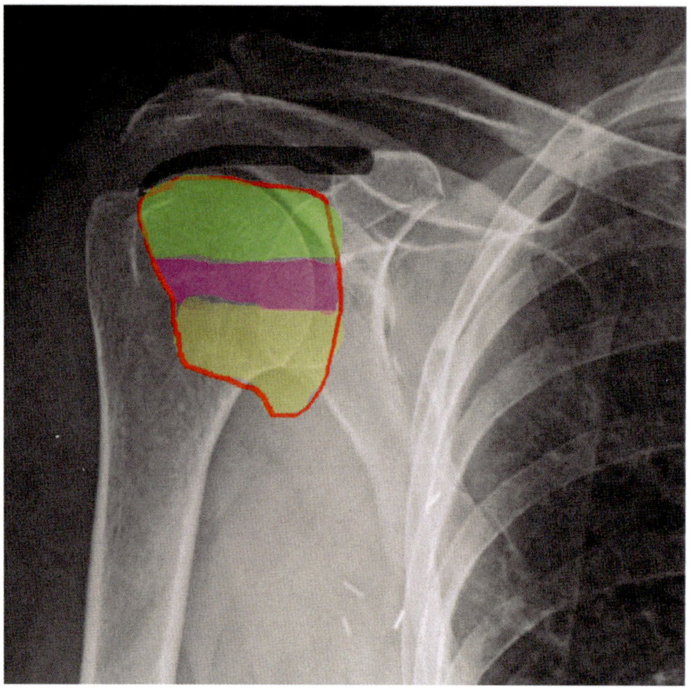

The rotator cuff, along with the long head of the biceps, stabilizes the glenohumeral joint actively (Figure 3). Paired contraction of the rotator cuff muscles holds the humeral head in close approximation to the glenoid cavity.

Figure 3: As seen from the front of the body, the subscapularis (red), supraspinatus (blue) and long head of the biceps (green) all dynamically stabilize the glenohumeral joint. (On the posterior side, the infra-spinatus and teres minor, not shown, provide stability as well.)

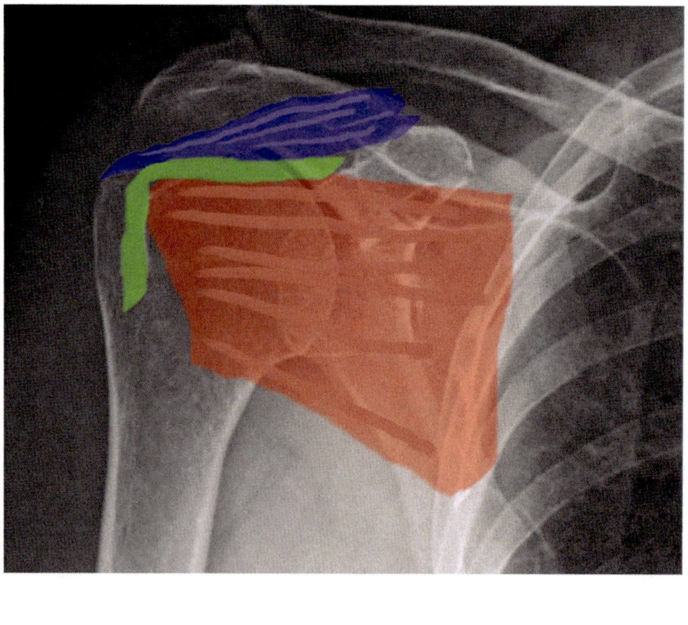

The axillary nerve is often injured with shoulder dislocations. The axillary nerve wraps around the surgical neck of the humerus and runs below the humeral head.

PATIENT PRESENTATION

A thorough history is essential to characterize a patient's shoulder instability. The patient may recall a specific traumatic instability event. Alternatively, the patient may have numerous incomplete instability events or describe generalized laxity of both shoulders or other joints.

Anterior instability often follows an injury to the arm when it is abducted and externally rotated. In contrast, posterior instability is often caused by a force applied to the arm when it is adducted, flexed and internally rotated. Inferior instability is associated with a history of instability with carrying heavy loads. Although anterior instability is the most common form, inferior, posterior and multidirectional instability must be considered.

With an acute anterior shoulder dislocation, the patient typically presents with the arm held closely at the side. Any attempt to abduct or rotate the arm is resisted because of pain. There is loss of the normal contour of the deltoid. The humeral head itself may be seen or felt anterior to its normal position.

The acute presentation of posterior shoulder instability is more subtle. A lack of external rotation compared to the contralateral normal shoulder may be the only presenting sign.

The physical exam should begin with evaluation of the asymptomatic shoulder for comparison.

Two simple tests may be used even by inexperienced examiners to evaluate shoulder instability.

The sulcus sign can be elicited by applying longitudinal inferior traction of the humerus; that is, by pulling down on the patient's wrist with the arm held at the side. Excessive inferior displacement of the humerus relative to the lateral border of the acromion creates a sulcus and reflects laxity of the capsule, (Figure 4).

Figure 4: The sulcus sign. The examiner pulls down on the arm at the elbow. If there is laxity of the shoulder, an indentation on the skin, aka a "sulcus", will be seen between the acromion and the humeral head. (with permission of https://www.shoulderdoc.co.uk/article/798)

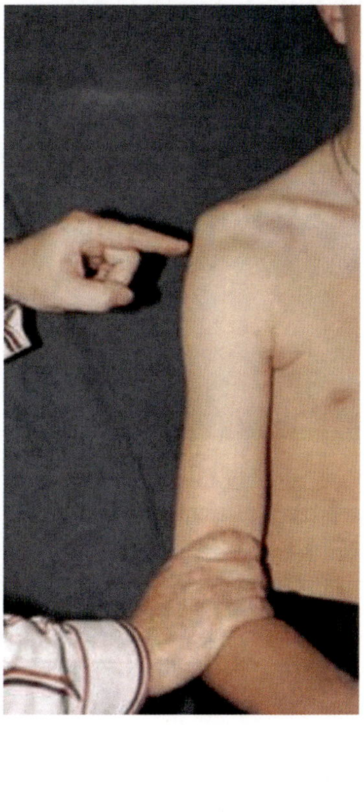

The anterior apprehension test is performed by asking the patient to abduct the shoulder (blue arrow) and externally rotate the arm (green curved arrow) – as if cocking the arm to throw a ball. A patient with anterior instability will be apprehensive in this position or might simply refuse to perform this maneuver (Figure 5).

Figure 5: The anterior apprehension test (see text).

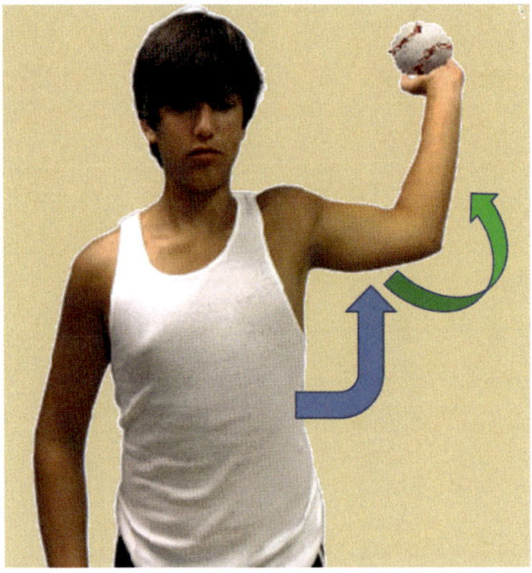

More subtle anterior instability can be detected by having the supine patient abduct the shoulder and externally rotate the arm, and the examiner can then push on the arm as if to glide the humeral head out of the joint.

Signs of generalized ligamentous laxity include the ability to touch the palms to the floor while bending at the waist; hyperextension of the elbows, metacarpophalangeal or knee joints; and the ability to abduct the thumb to the forearm. The presence of these so-called Beighton criteria is indicative of laxity.

OBJECTIVE EVIDENCE

To assess patients with suspected shoulder instability, obtain both an anteroposterior (AP) view (Figure 6) and an axillary lateral view of the shoulder. It is important to obtain two orthogonal views. A dislocated shoulder might look normal on the AP view and a dislocation may be missed if only this view is obtained.

Figure 6: Anterior shoulder dislocation. (Case courtesy of Dr Jeremy Jones, Radiopaedia.org, rID: 7132)

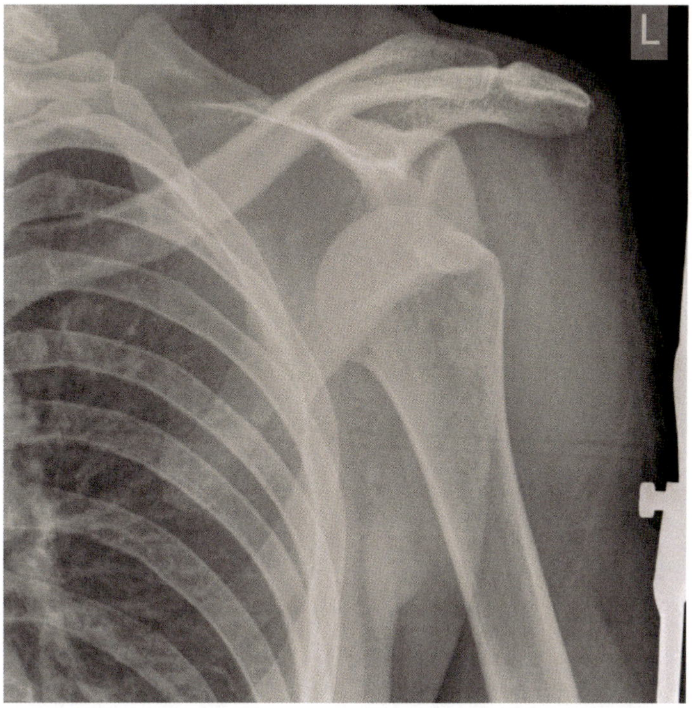

Magnetic resonance imaging (MRI) can be used to visualize the ligaments that might be torn with shoulder dislocation (Figure 7). MRI is more sensitive for the detection of labral injury if a contrast medium such as gadolinium is injected into the joint. MRI is especially useful for the evaluation of older patients with a dislocation as they are more likely to have torn the rotator cuff concurrently.

Figure 7: An MRI of the shoulder after reduction of a dislocation. Damage to the anterior labrum and edema within the humeral head, both caused by the dislocation, are noted with arrows. (Case courtesy of Dr. Mandakini Siwach, Radiopaedia.org, rID: 53957)

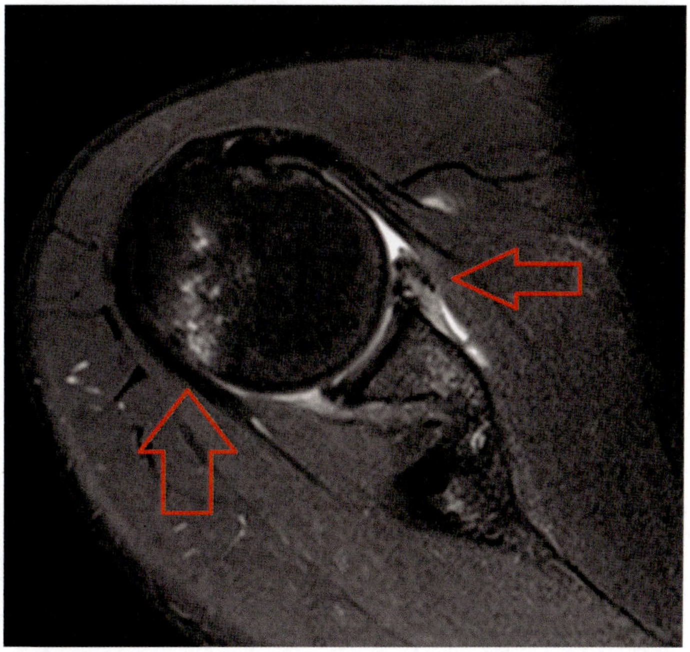

CT scans may be helpful for evaluation of the bony anatomy and should be obtained if there is suspicion of a large Hill-Sachs lesion or glenoid fracture.

EPIDEMIOLOGY

The annual incidence of shoulder dislocations in the United States is approximately 24 per 100,000 people. The incidence rates in military personnel and athletes are considerably higher. Anterior shoulder dislocations account for more than 95% of shoulder dislocations. Posterior dislocations account for about 4%, and inferior shoulder dislocations represent the remaining 1%.

Multidirectional shoulder instability is frequently bilateral. Its incidence peaks in young adulthood (approximately late teens) and is found especially in overhead athletes (pitchers, swimmers and gymnasts) or people with connective tissue disorders such as Ehlers-Danlos or Marfan's syndrome.

DIFFERENTIAL DIAGNOSIS

When patients present with suggested glenohumeral instability, physicians must exclude the following concomitant conditions:

- A Bankart lesion (avulsion of the anterior labrum),
- A "bony Bankart" lesion (a fracture of the anterior glenoid),
- A Hill Sachs defect (impaction fracture of the humeral head, caused by contact against the glenoid during dislocation),
- Fracture of the greater tuberosity (especially in older patients),
- Fracture of the lesser tuberosity (with posterior dislocation),
- Nerve injuries, especially axillary nerve,
- Generalized ligamentous laxity.

RED FLAGS

Seizures and electrocution can cause posterior shoulder dislocations and should be considered in any patients with that history and shoulder complaints. Likewise, the presence of a posterior shoulder dislocation raises the suspicion of an unreported seizure. Posterior shoulder dislocations are also associated with small lesser tuberosity fractures. These fractures might be missed if the films are not examined closely.

Multidirectional shoulder instability may suggest a connective tissue disorder such as Ehlers-Danlos or Marfan's syndrome.

Abnormal passive motion suggests that the shoulder is not reduced.

In patients older than 40 years, the orthopaedic surgeon should have a high index of suspicion for a concomitant rotator cuff tear.

Although axillary nerve injuries are seen in only a small minority of cases, they are frequent enough (~5% of cases) that the presence of dislocation itself is a "red flag" for a nerve injury and must be excluded on exam.

TREATMENT OPTIONS AND OUTCOMES

Acute shoulder dislocations should be reduced expeditiously. Any of a variety of reduction techniques can be performed. The Hippocratic method for anterior dislocations uses gentle longitudinal traction applied with a counterforce (e.g., a sheet placed in the patient's axilla). The Milch maneuver has the patient lying prone on the exam table with both abduction and external rotation forces applied to the arm as the physician's thumb attempts to push the humeral head into place.

Reduction is easiest when there is full relaxation of the shoulder musculature. Therefore, all attempts at reduction are best supplemented with either conscious sedation or an intra-articular anesthetic injection.

Radiographs after the procedure are required to verify reduction.

After reduction, a short period of immobilization is reasonable, followed by range of motion exercises and then a strengthening program.

Physical therapy alone may be adequate treatment for traumatic instability. Surgery may be considered especially in younger patients with a Bankart lesion or patients with a history of recurrent dislocations. Surgery is typically a repair of the capsule, along with a "shift" to tighten the tissue.

Patients with a shoulder dislocation are considered cleared to play when strength and full range of motion have returned to normal.

Multidirectional shoulder instability is treated with physical therapy – and then more physical therapy if that does not work. Operative stabilization is indicated only if instability that interferes with critical activities persists after extensive non-operative management.

Surgery for multidirectional shoulder instability attempts to plicate (that is, fold over and thereby tighten) the redundant capsular tissue. It is key that this plication is balanced, as too much tightening on one side (anteriorly, say) will just create more instability in the other direction.

The natural history of initial shoulder dislocations remains controversial. Recurrent dislocation is most strongly predicted by the age of the patient. In athletes younger than 20 years of age treated non-operatively, recurrence rates above 50% have been reported. Recurrent dislocation is less common in older patients, but in this cohort rotator cuff tears are more common and surgery may be needed to treat that aspect of the injury.

Athletes who have had a shoulder stabilization procedure after traumatic dislocation report a far lower dislocation recurrence rate (less than 15%) than would be expected from non-operative treatment. Most patients also report excellent subjective and objective clinical outcome scores.

RISK FACTORS AND PREVENTION

Patients might be at increased risk for shoulder instability for reasons under one's control (choice of sports, for example) or for reasons beyond individual control (abnormal glenoid anatomy and ligamentous laxity, to name two).

Even if there are non-modifiable risk factors, the odds of a dislocation may be minimized by assuring adequate strength of all muscles crossing the shoulder (including scapular-stabilizing muscles) and by keeping repetitive shoulder stress to a minimum.

MISCELLANY

Hippocrates not only invented a method of reducing the shoulder (Figure 8), he also devised a means of repairing the tissue injured by dislocation: namely, burning the capsule with a hot poker placed in the axilla. This method is frowned upon by modern authorities.

Figure 8: Hippocrates' method of reducing a dislocation of the shoulder. (https://en.wikipedia.org/wiki/Hippocrates#/media/File:GreekReduction.jpg)

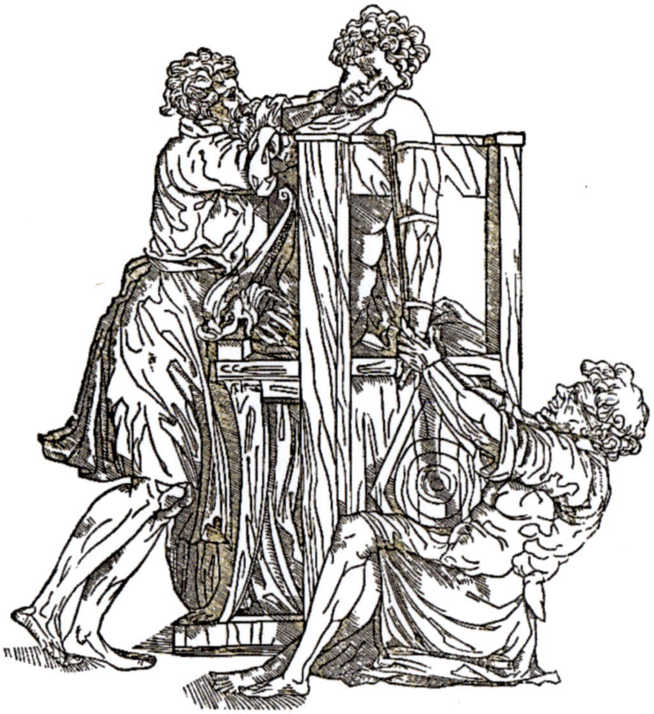

KEY TERMS

Glenohumeral instability, anterior dislocation, posterior dislocation, inferior dislocation, subluxation, humeral head, labrum, Bankart lesion, Hill-Sachs defect

SKILLS

Recognize history and signs suggesting dislocation. Recognize dislocation on imaging, and in particular, whether imaging is inadequate.

CHAPTER 10.

DISORDERS OF THE GLENOID LABRUM

DESCRIPTION

The glenoid labrum is a fibrocartilaginous rim attached around the margin of the glenoid cavity that serves to deepen the cavity. (The glenoid fossa of the scapula is relatively shallow, contacting at most only a third of the head of the humerus). The labrum is triangular in shape with a broad base and is fixed to the glenoid tapering to a thin free edge. The tendon of the long head of the biceps brachii blends with the labrum at the apex of the glenoid. Labral tears may result from acute injury, especially when the humeral head dislocates or subluxates, but also from traction via the biceps. Many labral tears are degenerative and are discovered incidentally on MRI.

STRUCTURE AND FUNCTION

The major shoulder joint is the glenohumeral joint, at which the humeral head articulates with the glenoid cavity (fossa or socket). Because the humeral head is larger than the fossa – the socket covers only a quarter of the humeral head – it is not very stable. To augment stability, a circumferential rim of fibrocartilaginous tissue attaches to the glenoid fossa and thereby increases the contact between the two sides of the joint (Figure 1).

Figure 1: A schematic drawing of a lateral view of the shoulder and an annotated lateral view x-ray highlight the glenoid fossa in green, the labrum in yellow and the biceps origin in red. To locate lesions of the labrum, the glenoid has been likened to a clock face, with the bicep's point of origin designated as the "12 O'clock position." (Modified from: https://en.wikipedia.org/wiki/Glenoid_labrum and https://radiopaedia.org/cases/48080)

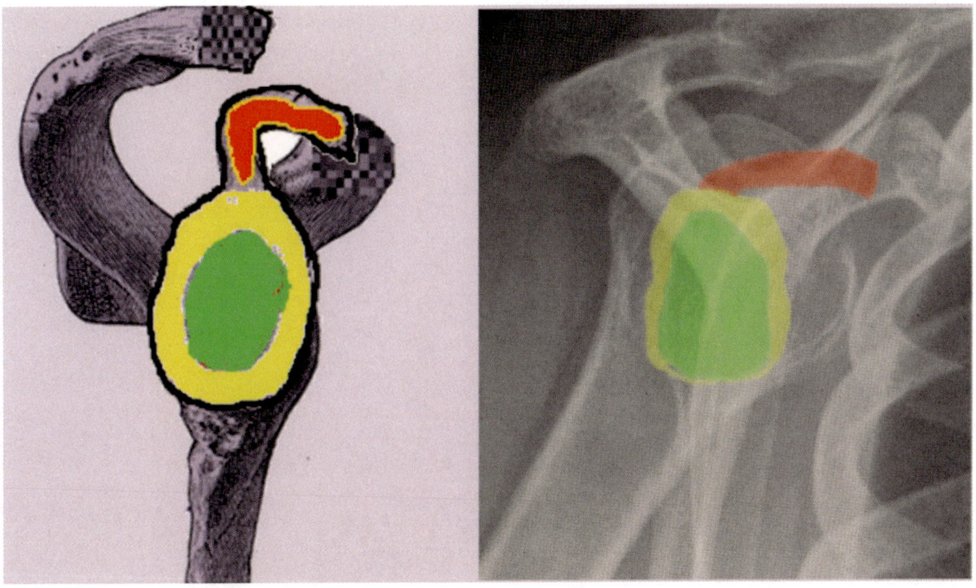

The labrum may be torn acutely, as in a traumatic anterior shoulder dislocation. Anterior dislocations often cause an avulsion of the anterior labrum, called a Bankart lesion.

There are two main theories to explain sub-acute tearing of the labrum. The first theory suggests that if the humeral head starts to subluxate (as it might tend to do, for example, if the capsule were lax), the biceps tendon would contract to constrain the humerus. Such repetitive contraction stretches the superior glenoid labrum. A second theory proposes that repeated motion results in cyclical compression and microtrauma to the labrum directly.

When a labral tear is above the "equator" of the glenoid it is called a SLAP tear: Superior Labrum, Anterior to Posterior.

SLAP tears are common among athletes playing a sport with high force overhead arm motion (e.g. tennis players and baseball pitchers).

A posteriorly directed force with the arm in a flexed, internally rotated and adducted position, e.g. weightlifters' bench press or football line blocking, can damage the posterior labrum

The proximal biceps tendon can also tear, independent of the labrum. The long head of the biceps is vulnerable to tearing, as it makes sharp turns as it courses out of the shoulder joint and down the arm. Tears are more common if there is stenosis of the bicipital groove or if there is a rotator cuff tear (perhaps placing additional demands on the biceps as a humeral head depressor).

PATIENT PRESENTATION

Acute tears are associated with overt trauma, such as falling hard onto an outstretched arm.

The symptoms of sub-acute labral tears include non-specific deep shoulder pain, a sense of catching or locking (due to a flap of loose cartilage), and perceived instability (which may or may not be reproduced on exam). There may be non-specific symptoms such as decreased range of motion or loss of strength. Symptoms tend to be aggravated with reaching overhead or across one's body.

No single physical sign or test has been shown to have both great sensitivity and specificity for SLAP tears. In O'Brien's active compression test, the patient stands upright with the affected arm flexed 90° and adducted 15° medial to the sagittal plane of the body. With the arm internally rotated, the examiner pushes the arm downward. The test is then repeated with the forearm in maximal supination. A positive test result is recorded when pain elicited by the first maneuver is decreased by the second maneuver (Figure 2).

Figure 2: O'Brien's test by having the patient elevate the arm to 90° and adduct 15° across the body. With the patient's arm internally rotated/pronated (thumb pointing down), the examiner pushes the arm downward (arrow). The test is deemed positive if this force is more painful than the same force applied with the patient's arm supinated.

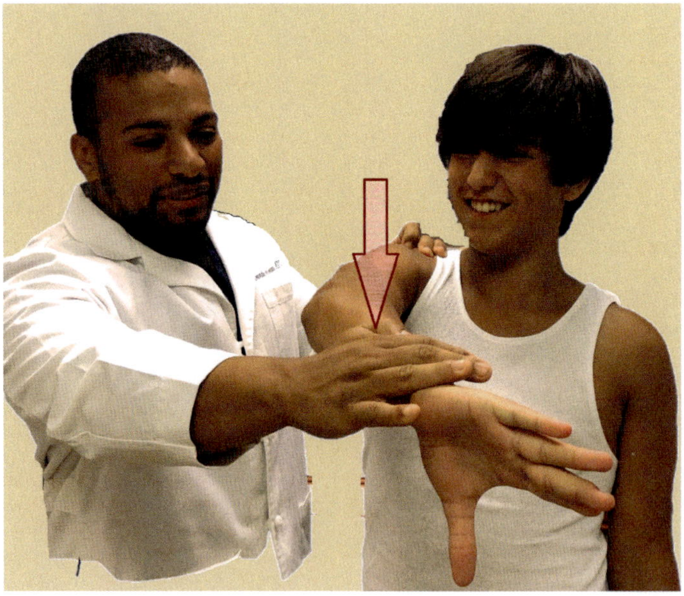

Isolated degenerative disease of the proximal biceps tendon presents with symptoms similar to rotator cuff disorders, but with the pain sometimes located in the bicipital groove.

Speed test's (Figure 3) is positive when there is pain in the proximal biceps produced with forward elevation of the shoulder with the elbow extended and forearm supinated. Yergason's test (Figure 4) will produce pain in the biceps groove when a patient with biceps pathology attempts to actively supinate against the examiner's resistance.

Figure 3: Speed test's is performed by applying resistance (blue arrow) when the patient attempts forward elevation of the shoulder, with the elbow extended and forearm supinated. Pain in the bicipital groove (black star) near the shoulder is a positive response.

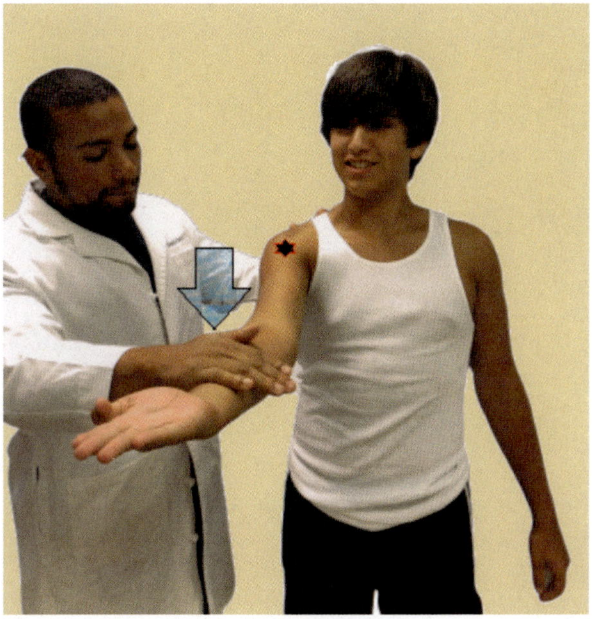

Figure 4: To perform Yergason's test, the patient and examiner start in the handshake position. The patient then attempts to supinate (blue arrow) the arm (turning palm facing upward) against the examiner's resistance. Pain localizing to the bicipital groove (black arrow) is a positive response.

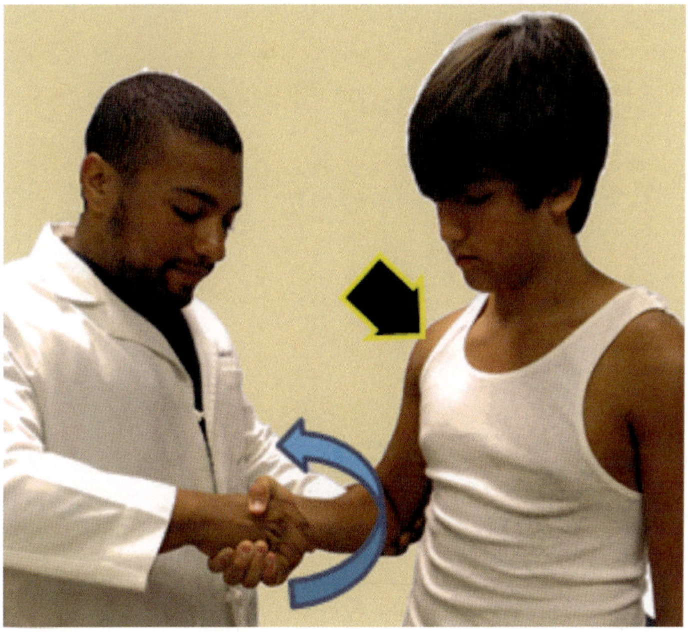

OBJECTIVE EVIDENCE

Because the labrum and proximal biceps are soft tissues, they are not seen on plain radiography. Accordingly, x-rays are often not informative when these structures are damaged.

MRI can be diagnostic for labral tears (Figure 5), but both sensitivity and specificity increases with the injection of contrast (creating a so-called MRI-arthrogram).

Figure 5: An MRI showing a superior labral tear. The labrum should be a dark triangle throughout; here there is a faint line at the base of the triangle, where the labrum attaches to the glenoid. (from https://openorthopaedicsjournal.com/VOLUME/12/PAGE/314/FULLTEXT/)

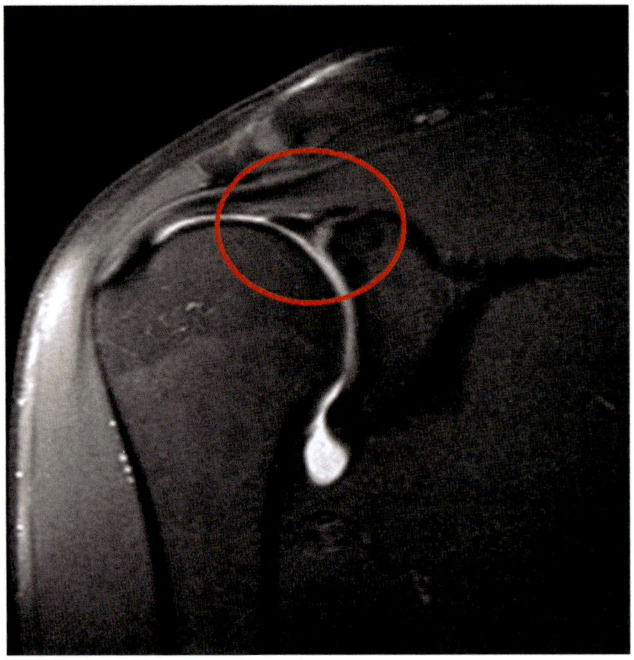

A conventional MRI might show an associated paralabral cyst (Figure 6), offering a hint that there is a labral tear (that is not seen explicitly).

Figure 6: An MRI showing a labral cyst (red arrow), suggestive of a tear. (from https://openorthopaedicsjournal.com/VOLUME/12/PAGE/314/FULLTEXT/)

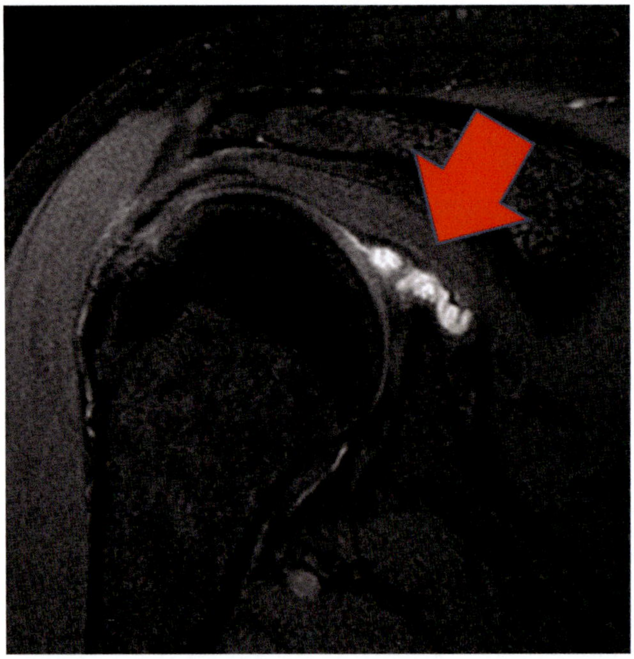

EPIDEMIOLOGY

There are no firm data on the prevalence of labral disorders, because many people do not seek medical care. It is known that starting at about age of 35, the superior labrum is less firmly attached to the glenoid, leading to anterior-superior rim tears, and that at about age 60 internal age-related degenerative changes are more common.

DIFFERENTIAL DIAGNOSIS

The main competing diagnoses (which may be present concurrently) are rotator cuff tears or degeneration and shoulder instability.

RED FLAGS

There are no particular red flag diagnoses for the symptoms associated with labral disorders.

TREATMENT OPTIONS AND OUTCOMES

Initial treatment options for a torn labrum generally include the use of nonsteroidal anti-inflammatory drugs (NSAIDs) and a period of rest. Physical therapy is then initiated to strengthen the rotator cuff muscles.

Surgical intervention depends on the type of labral lesion, but an arthroscopic repair is most commonly used (Figure 7). Frayed labral tears are treated with debridement.

Figure 7: Arthroscopic view of a labral tear (red line) before and after repair. (Courtesy of Fotios Tjoumakaris, MD)

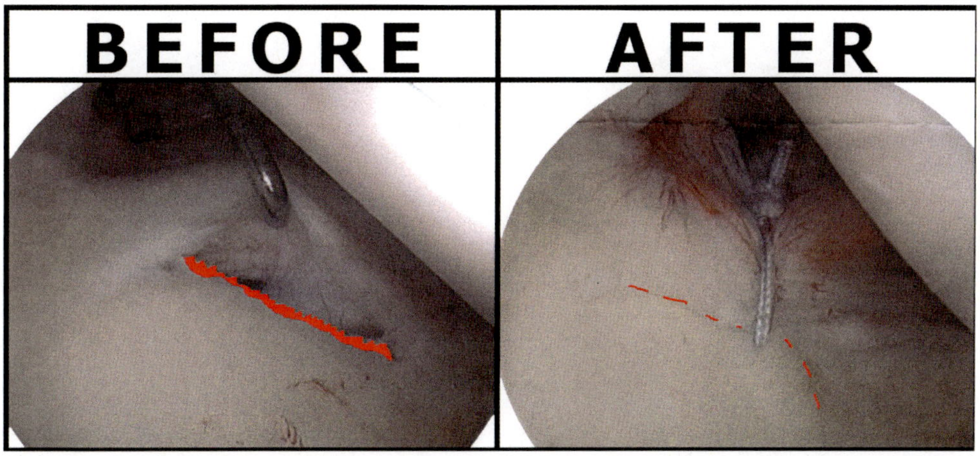

Damage to the biceps anchor can be treated with arthroscopic fixation of the superior labrum, but patients 45 years of age or older are prone to stiffness if the tear is repaired. Accordingly, fixation is considered relatively contraindicated in these patients.

Proximal biceps tendinopathy is also first treated with NSAIDs and therapy. A steroid injection near, but not in, the tendon may be helpful. Should that not work, surgical release (tenotomy) or repair to the humerus (tenodesis) may be chosen. Tenotomy may cause an asymmetric bulging of the biceps in the affected arm. Tenodesis may be associated with pain in the bicipital groove. This complication may be prevented by attaching the tendon to the bone in a more inferior position, i.e. in the sub-pectoral region of the humerus.

Most patients with labral tears will return to their pre-injury level of shoulder function, with slightly worse results seen among overhead throwing athletes.

The most common overt complication for surgical treatment is an injury to nerves around the shoulder, but this is rare (less than 1% of cases) and usually resolves within 6 weeks.

Some patients, especially older ones, have lost motion, though this may be ameliorated with therapy once the tissue repair has healed.

RISK FACTORS AND PREVENTION

The main risk factors for labral disorders are sports demanding repetitive overhead motion (baseball, tennis, swimming) and increasing age (due to degenerative changes in the tissue as well as risk of falls).

These risk factors are not really amenable to change, but strengthening of the rotator cuff muscles, adequate warm-up before activity, and adequate rest intervals between episodes of intense activity can all be defended as common sense.

MISCELLANY

About 1% of people have a congenital glenoid labrum variant where the anterosuperior labrum is absent. This variant is known as a "Buford complex".

KEY TERMS

Labrum, SLAP lesion, Bankart lesion, rotator cuff, arthroscopy, torn biceps

SKILLS

Categorize MRI findings of a torn labrum. Perform physical exam to identify labral pathology.

CHAPTER 11.

DISORDERS OF THE BICEPS AND THE TRICEPS

DESCRIPTION

The biceps and the triceps are the major muscles of the upper arm. Both muscles take origin from the humerus itself but also have an origin on the scapula; both insert on the forearm, namely, the radius and ulna respectively. Distally, both muscles are susceptible to overuse and strain, and may rupture or avulse from their insertions. Rupture of the biceps and triceps are most commonly due to increased eccentric force through a degenerated tendon. Common proximal biceps conditions include tendonitis, subluxation and rupture of the long head of the biceps tendon, which takes origin from the supraglenoid tubercle of the scapula (and is therefore primarily a shoulder muscle). Proximal triceps disease is rare.

STRUCTURE AND FUNCTION

As its name implies, the biceps (Figure 1) has two proximal divisions. The long head of the biceps brachii originates from the glenoid labrum at the supraglenoid tubercle; the short head from the coracoid process. The biceps inserts at the radial tuberosity. It is supplied by the brachial artery and is innervated by the musculocutaneous nerve.

Figure 1: Anterior view of the biceps, with the long head in red and the short head in green. (from https://en.wikipedia.org/wiki/Biceps)

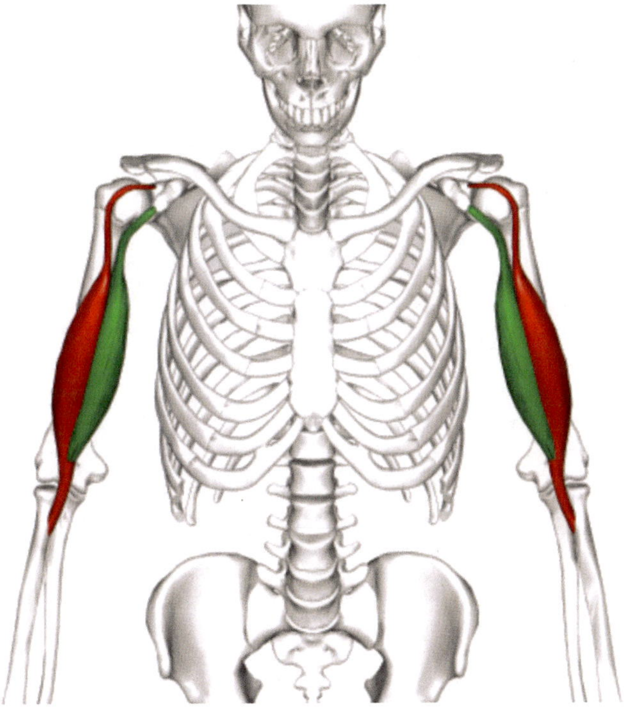

The biceps flexes the elbow, but perhaps contrary to popular belief, it is not the most powerful flexor of the forearm– a role which actually belongs to the deeper brachialis muscle. Indeed, when the forearm is in pronation (the palm faces the ground), there is only a minimal contribution from the biceps brachii to elbow flexion (Figure 2). In this position, the main flexor of the elbow is the brachialis, with contributions from the brachioradialis and supinator as well.

The biceps brachii functions primarily as a supinator of the forearm (turning the palm upwards). This action, which is aided by the supinator muscle, requires the elbow to be at least partially flexed. If the elbow is fully extended, supination is then primarily carried out by the supinator muscle.

Figure 2: With the forearm in the pronated position (left), flexing the elbow will contract the biceps, but only with the forearm in a supinated position (right) does the biceps fully contract to its minimum length (and maximal bulge). (Modified from https://en.wikipedia.org/wiki/Biceps)

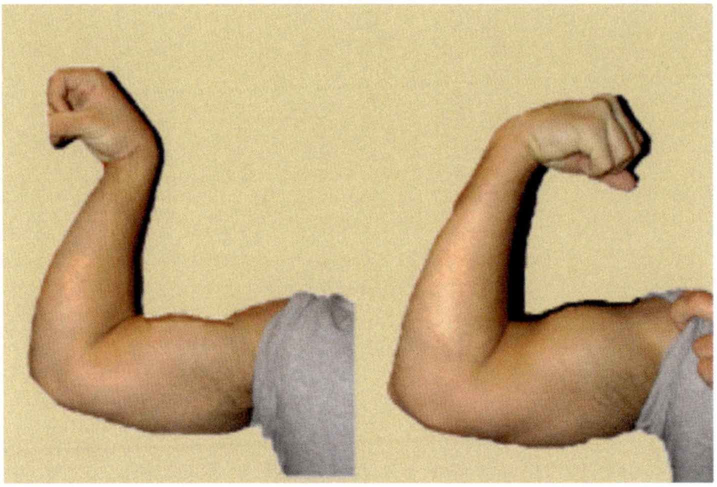

The triceps has three proximal divisions known as "heads": two which originate from the posterior humerus, the lateral head and medial head; and one, the long head, which originates from the infraglenoid tubercle of the scapula (Figure 3). These then blend together and insert on the olecranon process of the ulna. The triceps is an extensor muscle of the elbow joint and is an antagonist of the biceps and brachialis muscles. It can also fixate the elbow joint – that is, hold it in a fixed position – when the forearm and hand are used for fine movements. The triceps is supplied by the deep brachial artery and posterior circumflex humeral artery and is innervated by the radial nerve.

Figure 3: Posterior view of the triceps, with long head in red, lateral head in yellow and medial head (deep and obscured mostly) in green. (from https://en.wikipedia.org/wiki/Triceps)

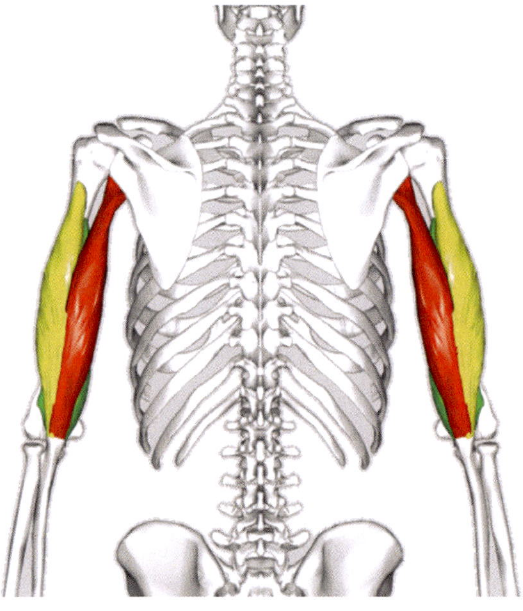

PATIENT PRESENTATION

Patients with a distal biceps rupture present after experiencing a painful pop in the elbow after an eccentric force is applied – that is, as the elbow is moved from flexion into extension by an external force, with the biceps attempting to resist or slow that motion.

Patients will complain of pain and weakness, primarily in supination.

The physical exam reveals tenderness to palpation and possibly a defect, with some proximal retraction of the muscle belly as well, causing a "reverse Popeye sign." Ecchymosis in the antecubital fossa may be seen too.

The hook test may reveal the absence of the normal tendon insertion (Figure 4). In this test, the examiner's index finger attempts to pluck or "hook" the biceps tendon in the fossa, with the patient actively flexing the elbow and supinating the forearm.

Figure 4: The hook test. When the biceps tendon is intact, the examiner's finger can grasp (or "hook") the lateral edge of the biceps tendon. An absence of any "hookable" tendon suggests a rupture.

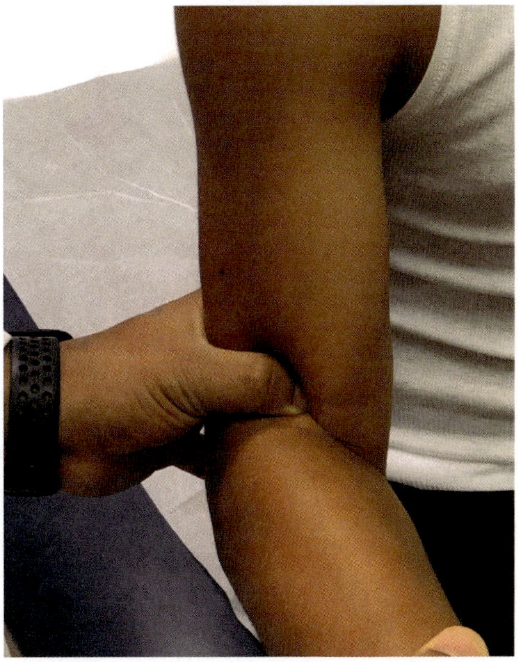

Patients with a distal triceps rupture likewise present after a painful pop, usually after a fall. (When a patient lands on the outstretched hand, there may be a force tending to collapse, or flex, the elbow. The triceps can be injured as it resists this force.)

The physical exam of a patient with a triceps injury usually reveals painful swelling and ecchymosis over the posterior aspect of the elbow. Here too there may be a palpable defect. An inability to extend the elbow against resistance suggests the diagnosis, though a partial tear may allow some motion, or may be so painful that no motion is seen (despite having some tendon in continuity). Therefore, a modified Thompson squeeze test (similar to what is done in the calf for suspected Achilles ruptures), in which the triceps muscle is firmly squeezed with the patient lying prone and the arm hanging off the edge of the table, may be performed: a lack of any elbow motion with this maneuver suggests complete disruption of triceps.

OBJECTIVE EVIDENCE

Plain radiographs will reveal any fracture; there may also be a flake of bone seen with avulsions.

MRI can be used to differentiate partial from complete rupture and to evaluate the degree of retraction.

EPIDEMIOLOGY

Distal biceps tendonitis is relatively rare; proximal lesions are far more common, representing approximately 90% of biceps tears. Tendonitis and subluxation of the long head are very common, often seen alongside degenerative rotator cuff tears in older patients.

Ruptures of the distal biceps occur most commonly at the point of insertion, either as a complete or partial avulsion from the radial tuberosity. This is an almost-exclusively male condition, and almost always seen in the dominant arm.

Ruptures of the triceps are rare (about 1% of all tendon ruptures) and affect males in a 2 to 1 ratio. This condition is typically found in weightlifters and body builders.

Patients with ruptures of either tendon are usually in the age of 30 to 50: old enough to have degenerative change, but young enough to exercise vigorously enough to cause damage.

DIFFERENTIAL DIAGNOSIS

Complete ruptures of the distal biceps tendon and triceps tendon should be differentiated from incomplete ruptures, as this may dictate whether surgical or non-operative management is indicated.

An inability to move the elbow might reflect a bone injury, which would be detected or excluded on radiographs.

RED FLAGS

Tendon rupture might signify use of steroids and other banned substances. Falls in the elderly may signify underlying disease (and risk of further falls).

TREATMENT OPTIONS AND OUTCOMES

Patients with a distal biceps rupture are indicated for surgical repair if the injury imposes significant functional loss. Even with a distal biceps rupture, most of elbow flexion is preserved as the biceps is not the main flexor. The main residual weakness will be with supination; and surgery is chosen with that in mind.

Non-operative treatment usually results in up to 50% lost supination strength, but only about 30% loss of flexion strength.

Operative repair (Figure 5) is either with an anterior single or double incision technique using both an anterior incision to prepare the tendon and a second posterior-lateral one to fix the tendon to the bone. The single incision surgery reduces the risk of heterotopic ossification but with higher risk of nerve injury.

Figure 5: The biceps tendon prepared for surgical reattachment into a socket on the radius is shown (photo A). A small metallic button is placed on the end of the tendon, to lock on the opposite surface of the radius (See diagram B) (Courtesy https://openorthopaedicsjournal.com/VOLUME/11/PAGE/1364/FULLTEXT/)

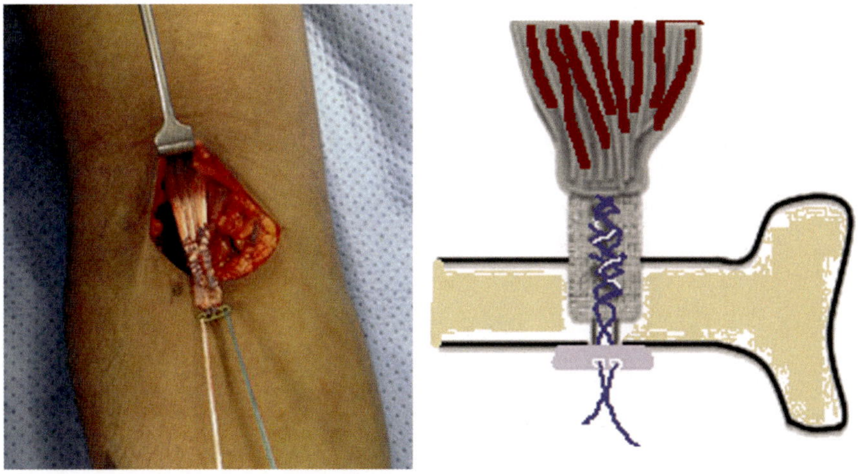

(The nerves at risk are the lateral antebrachial cutaneous and the radial nerve; injury to the former is more common, to the latter more severe.)

Patients with a complete distal triceps rupture are typically indicated for surgical repair. The patients are immobilized for only about 2 weeks post-operatively (to minimize contracture of the elbow) with active range of motion initiated shortly thereafter. Non-operative treatment with splint immobilization can be chosen if only a partial tear is present (demonstrated by an ability to extend against gravity) or if the patient has low demands and is too sick for surgery.

The patient reported outcomes following distal biceps and triceps rupture repairs are generally very good, however, there is the potential for significant complications. Following distal biceps tendon repairs, nerve damage, re-rupture, and heteropic ossifications can be seen. Elbow stiffness, ulnar nerve injury, and re-rupture are the most common complications following triceps tendon repair, although these generally occur in less than 10% of patients.

RISK FACTORS AND PREVENTION

Risk factors for acute ruptures include excessive weightlifting, anabolic steroids, renal disease, fluoroquinolone use, and smoking.

MISCELLANY

The "Popeye" sign is named after the cartoon character due to the characteristic bulge of the muscle, yet interestingly, Popeye himself had meager biceps; his muscle mass was mostly in the forearm (see Figure 6).

Figure 6: The real Popeye did not have a "Popeye" sign.

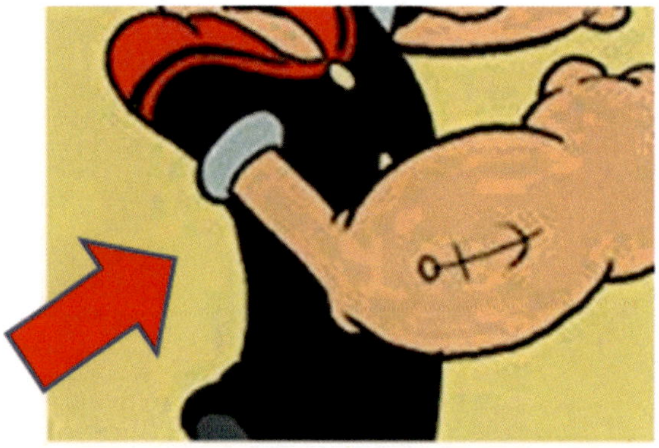

As many bodybuilders know, the triceps accounts for approximately 60 percent of the upper arm's muscle mass; thus exercising this muscle, and not the biceps, is apt to produce larger arms.

KEY TERMS

Biceps, triceps, tendonitis, rupture

SKILLS

Physical examination to diagnose disorders of the biceps and triceps.

CHAPTER 12.

DISORDERS OF THE ELBOW LIGAMENTS

DESCRIPTION

The elbow joint is stabilized by the ulnar (medial) collateral ligament, the lateral collateral ligament, and the annular ligament. The ligaments provide valgus and varus stability, and allow for rotation, respectively. Additional static stability is provided by the capsule. Each of these ligaments can be injured by elbow trauma or overuse. Injuries of the ulnar collateral ligament are prevalent in overhead throwing athletes due to the high stresses on the elbow as the arm accelerates. Injuries to the lateral collateral ligament are often the result of acute high energy trauma (such as an elbow dislocation). Injuries to the annular ligament are rare, but in children under the age of 5, a sharp tug on the arm may allow the annular ligament to slide over the head of the radius and get caught in the elbow joint, a condition known as "Nursemaid's Elbow".

STRUCTURE AND FUNCTION

The ulnar collateral ligament (Figure 1) is composed of three bundles (the anterior, posterior, and transverse) and is the primary elbow stabilizer against valgus stress. The anterior bundle is the main stabilizer of the ulna from 30 to 120 degrees of elbow motion. The posterior bundle provides stability at higher degrees of flexion. The transverse bundle is thought to have no significant role in elbow stabilization. From 0 to 30 degrees of elbow motion, the joint is stabilized by bony congruity.

Figure 1: Annotated x-rays showing the ligaments of the elbow. At left, is a view from the lateral side. The annular ligament is red, the lateral ulnar collateral ligament is black, and the radial collateral ligament is purple. In the center panel, an AP view with the ulnar collateral ligament in green, the annular ligament in red and the radial collateral ligament in purple is shown. In the panel at right a medial sided view is shown, with the anterior bundle of the ulnar collateral ligament in green and the posterior bundle in yellow. The transverse bundle is not shown. (X-rays courtesy of Dr. Bruno Di Muzio, Radiopaedia.org, rID: 44153)

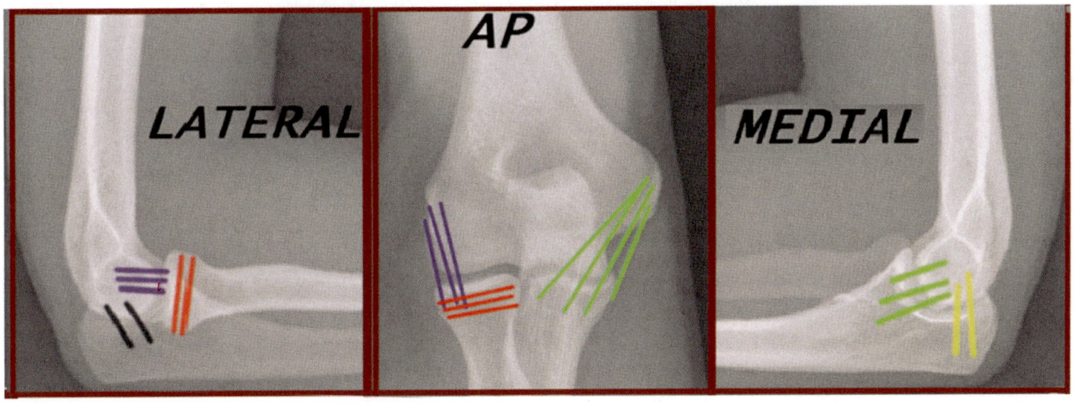

During the acceleration phase of a pitch, the elbow extends from approximately 110 degrees of flexion to 20 degrees. This generates a very high valgus force at the elbow and can produce small tears in the ligament.

The lateral collateral ligament is actually complex, including both a lateral radial collateral ligament and a lateral ulnar collateral ligament. The lateral ulnar collateral ligament is the primary stabilizer to varus stress. It originates on the lateral humeral epicondyle and inserts on the ulna.

Injury to the lateral collateral ligament is most often caused by an elbow dislocation.

As its name implies, the annular ligament forms a ring that surrounds the radial head, allowing the radius to twist relative to the ulna at the proximal radioulnar joint. This allows supination and pronation of the forearm.

PATIENT PRESENTATION

Injury to the ulnar collateral ligament can present as acute injury (classically, with a "pop" during a single pitch, associated with pain and difficulty throwing thereafter). It may also present as a chronic condition, manifested by an aching pain and decreased performance, including loss of velocity and control (accuracy). There may also be paresthesias reported in the ring and small fingers, due to traction on the ulnar nerve.

A focused patient history should include questions about the onset of pain, what the patient was doing when the pain started, sports played, and the frequency of participation.

On physical exam, palpation of the ulnar collateral ligament can help identify location of injury. Tenderness over the ulnar collateral ligament is a sensitive marker, but the specificity for ulnar collateral ligament tears is low.

Figure 2: The examiner's right index finger is on the patient's ulnar collateral ligament.

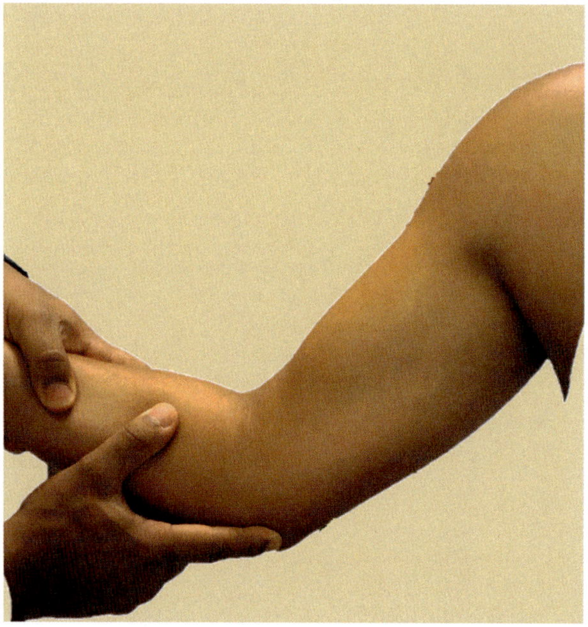

Medial elbow instability can be difficult to reproduce on exam, as it may be seen only with the high forces generated during throwing; the examiner's force will not reproduce the instability.

The valgus stress test is performed by passively placing the elbow in 30 degrees of flexion, and then externally rotating the humerus while applying a valgus stress.

Figure 3: The valgus stress test of the elbow. The examiner stabilizes the elbow with his or her upper hand, and then attempts to externally rotate the arm by applying a force to the wrist. This force is transmitted to the humerus via the ulnar collateral ligament and thus tests its integrity.

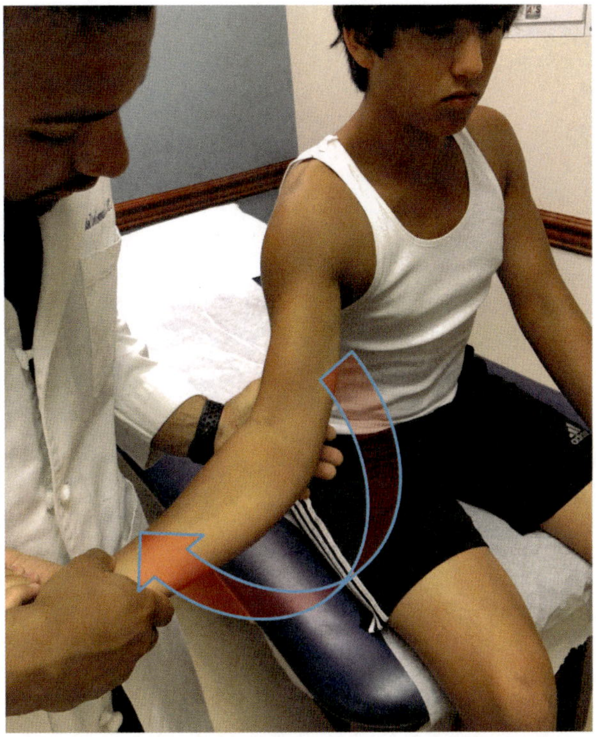

The "milking maneuver" creates a valgus stress on the elbow, by pulling on the patient's thumb with the forearm supinated and elbow flexed at 90 degrees. A positive test is noted by reported apprehension, though instability or pain may also be noted.

Figure 4: The "milking maneuver". Pulling down on the thumb when the elbow is supported, the forearm is supinated and elbow is flexed (as shown) creates a valgus force at the elbow. Needless to say, the examiner is the one to position the patient and apply the force. Here our talent model is performing the test on himself to demonstrate the maneuver without an examiner in front of the camera.

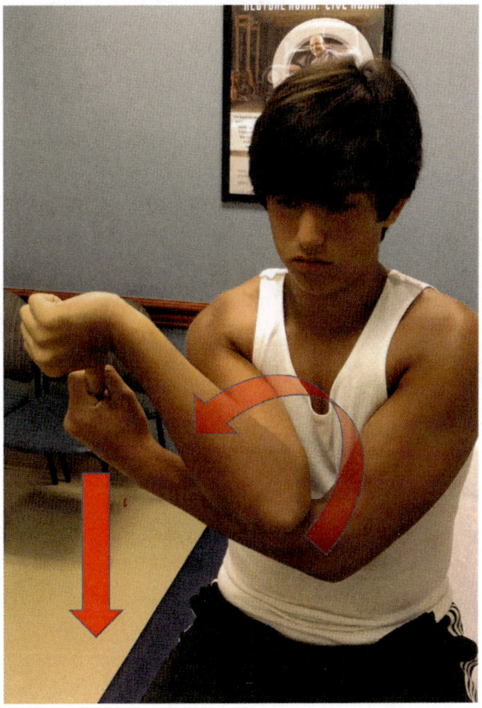

Late manifestations of lateral collateral ligament injuries include pain and mechanical symptoms. A report of symptoms specifically with resisted elbow extension, such as pushing off arm rests to get up from a chair, suggests a deficiency of the lateral collateral ligament with possible rotatory instability.

The physical exam is characterized by tenderness over the lateral collateral ligament, with varus instability seen on provocative testing.

One may elicit instability with the lateral pivot-shift test. The patient is instructed to hold the forearm in a supinated position and the examiner then applies a valgus stress to the elbow and, concurrently, passively flexes the elbow. This maneuver is difficult if the patient is awake or the examiner is inexperienced. It may be simpler to ask the patient to do a push-up maneuver with the forearm supinated, as in the pushing off a chair's armrests to arise from sitting. Pain, a sense of instability or the mere reluctance to attempt this suggest instability.

OBJECTIVE EVIDENCE

Radiographs may detect fracture (stress or acute), degenerative change, loose bodies or growth plate abnormalities. Radiographs should include AP and lateral views of the elbow; oblique views can help evaluate the olecranon osteophytes. Medial joint-line opening can demonstrate ligament failure, but stress views are not recommended, as they may worsen the condition.

Magnetic resonance imaging can show ulnar collateral ligament tears (Figure 5) or thickening of the ligament reflecting a chronic injury. Magnetic Resonance Arthrography can help differentiate between full-thickness and partial undersurface tears. MRI often shows edema in the flexor-pronator origin in addition to the torn ligament.

Figure 5: The arrow points to a distal medial collateral ligament avulsion. (from https://www.dovepress.com/article_metric.php?article_id=40434)

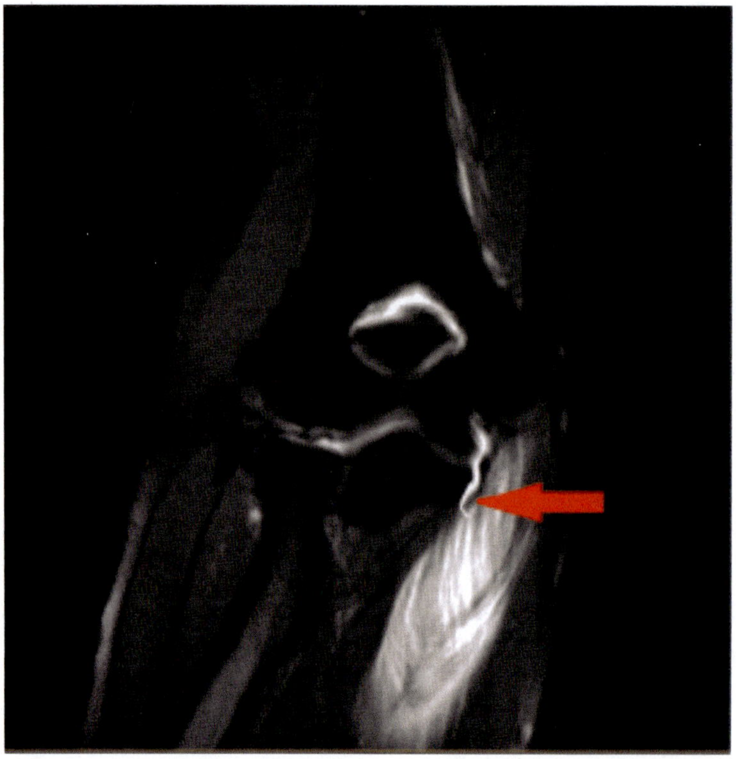

Magnetic Resonance Imaging is less effective for lateral collateral ligament tears; this diagnosis is made by history and physical examination, and may require examination under anesthesia for confirmation.

EPIDEMIOLOGY

Ulnar collateral ligament injuries can occur in individuals who routinely play sports that involve an overhead throwing motion including cricket, javelin, tennis or volleyball. It is commonly associated with professional American Baseball pitchers. More recent observational studies report a high incidence of injury in high-school-age-pitchers. A 5-year report from the NCAA Injury Surveillance Program reports overall incidence of ulnar collateral ligament injury to be 1.12 per 10,000 athletic exposures (N=20) with 85% of injury occurring during throwing.

Lateral collateral ligament injuries are rare.

DIFFERENTIAL DIAGNOSIS

The differential diagnosis for medial elbow pain (and generalized decline in pitching performance) includes medial epicondylitis, flexor-pronator injuries, ulnar neuropathy, apophysitis, posteromedial osteophytes, and stress fracture of the ulna.

RED FLAGS

Subtle complaints of ulnar collateral ligament dysfunction without any overt findings on exam may be considered a "red flag" for impending injury, especially if the symptoms are not respected and the patient (often a throwing athlete) continues to engage in provocative activities.

TREATMENT OPTIONS AND OUTCOMES

Young athletes with a partial tear of the ulnar collateral ligament are advised to not throw for four to six weeks. Thereafter, they should start a rehabilitation process that involves pitching mechanics, shoulder kinematics, and core, lower extremity, and upper extremity strengthening. Once the patient is pain free and kinetic deficits of the pitching mechanics have been addressed, the patient is gradually integrated into a throwing program.

The efficacy of platelet rich plasma injections has not been established.

Corticosteroid injections are not recommended because they may weaken the ligaments.

Surgical management of ulnar collateral ligament tears is reserved for high level throwing athletes with symptomatic instability. Direct repair of the ligament is not typically performed. Reconstruction of the ulnar collateral ligament is often performed with autograft from the ipsilateral palmaris longus (though only 85% of people have a palmaris longus muscle, and among those who do, the tendon may be too short. In those cases, reconstruction is performed with gracilis tendon graft.) Return to competitive throwing occurs 10 to 14 months post-operatively.

Acute care treatment of lateral collateral ligament injuries is dictated by the treatment of the elbow dislocation that is often its cause.

Chronic lateral collateral ligament deficiency is initially treated with bracing, strengthening, and activity modification. Failing that, reconstruction with a graft may be needed.

Reconstruction of the ulnar collateral ligament appears to be highly effective. Return to an equal or higher level of play has been reported to be as high as 90%. A 2014 study of 41 professional baseball pitchers reported no significant differences in pitch velocity and common performance measurements between players who returned to play after ulnar collateral ligament reconstruction and pair-matched controls. (It is not clear to what extent the one-year hiatus and rehabilitation plays in this.)

Surgery for chronic lateral collateral ligament deficiency is likewise effective: the recurrence rate for instability is less than 10%.

RISK FACTORS AND PREVENTION

Risk factors for ulnar collateral ligament injury include overuse of overhead throwing, particularly in youth pitchers. Recent trends amongst youth athletes have transformed baseball into more of a year-round sport. An epidemiology study from the American Sports Medicine Institute notes that pitch count is correlated with elbow and shoulder pain in pitchers. Youth pitchers should be limited to under 100 innings pitched per calendar year as risk of serious injury is 3.5 times greater above this limit. Limiting pitch count and not pitching year-round is probably more important than avoiding certain pitch type (fastballs vs curveballs, etc.).

MISCELLANY

Reconstruction of the ulnar collateral ligament was first performed in 1974. This surgery was performed by Dr. Frank Jobe on an American professional baseball player named Tommy John. These days, the procedure is known by many as "Tommy John Surgery".

KEY TERMS

ulnar collateral ligament of the elbow, lateral collateral ligament, varus and valgus stress test of the elbow, milking maneuver, ulnar collateral Tommy John Surgery, ulnar collateral ligament reconstruction

SKILLS

Recognizing collateral ligament disorders on examination and imaging.

CHAPTER 13.

OSTEOCHONDRAL INJURIES OF THE ELBOW

DESCRIPTION

Throwing places extremely high stresses on the elbow and thus overuse can damage the articular (cartilage) surfaces. Two characteristic areas are affected in throwing athletes: the olecranon process of the ulna and the distal humerus where it articulates with the radius, namely, the capitellum. In the olecranon, valgus forces erode the surface cartilage, and stimulate the production of bone spurs. In the distal humerus, more often the inciting pathology is ischemia of the subchondral bone causing osteonecrosis, a condition known as osteochondritis dissecans. Most patients with chondral injuries to the elbow recover with rest, but surgery may be needed if there are loose bodies or unstable cartilage flaps.

STRUCTURE AND FUNCTION

The elbow joint consists of the distal end of the humerus and the proximal aspects of the radius and ulna; and has three articulations: the ulnohumeral articulation, the radiohumeral articulation (also known as the radiocapitellar joint) and the proximal radioulnar joint (See Figures 1, 2 and 3).

Figure 1: The three joints of the elbow: the ulnohumeral (red), radiocapitellar (blue) and proximal radioulnar (green).

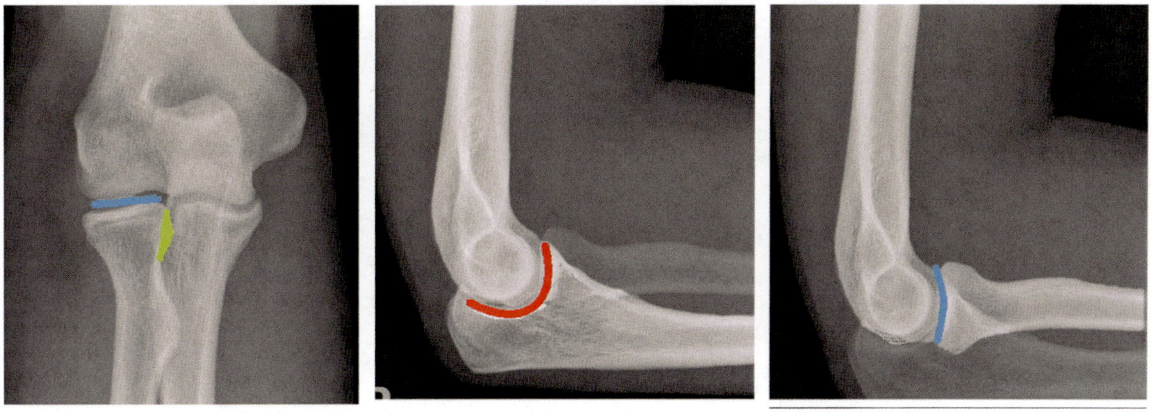

Figure 2: The bones and landmarks of the elbow joint seen on AP view. KEY: 1. Lateral supracondylar ridge; 2. Medial supracondylar ridge; 3. Olecranon fossa; 4. Medial epicondyle; 5. Lateral epicondyle; 6. Capitellum; 7. Olecranon; 8. Trochlea; 9. Coronoid process of ulna; 10. Proximal radioulnar joint; 11. Head of radius; 12. Neck of radius; 13. Tuberosity of radius; 14. Ulna. (courtesy www.orthopaedicsone.com)

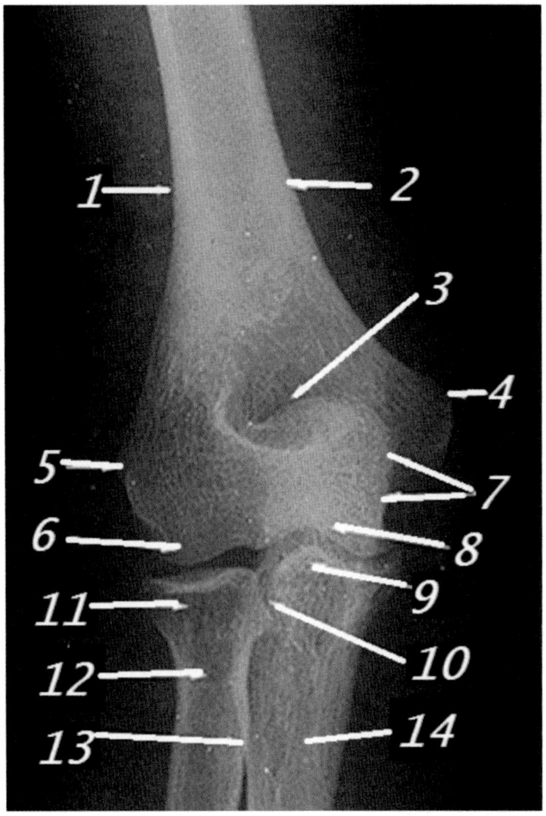

Figure 3: The bones and landmarks of the elbow joint seen on Lateral view. KEY: 1. Supracondylar ridge; 2. Trochlea; 3. Olecranon; 4. Trochlear notch; 5. Coronoid process of ulna; 6. Head of radius; 7. Neck of radius; 8. Tuberosity of radius; 9. Ulna. (courtesy www.orthopaedicsone.com)

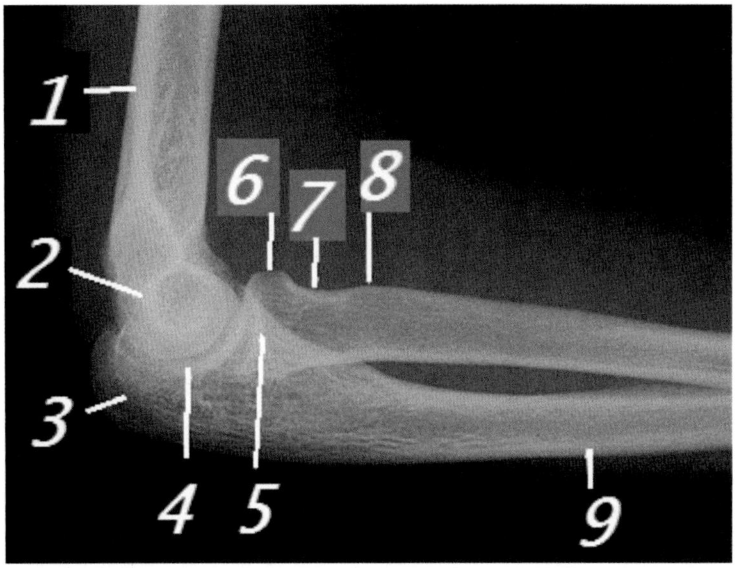

The ulnohumeral joint consists of the olecranon and the coronoid process of the ulna articulating with the humerus at the trochlea. The primary function/motion of the ulnohumeral joint is flexion and extension of the elbow.

A so-called valgus extension overload injury can result from excessive forces in the elbow during the throwing motion and is characterized by the breakdown of cartilage on the olecranon.

The radiocapitellar joint is the articulation of the proximal radius (radial head) with the distal end of the humerus (capitellum) and functions to pronate and supinate the lower arm. The radiocapitellar joint is supplied by the radial recurrent and interosseous recurrent arteries. This blood supply can be too-easily disrupted by repetitive microtrauma leading to ischemia and osteonecrosis. The constellation of necrosis and disruption of the joint surface is called osteochondritis dissecans. Osteochondrosis of the capitellum in patients under ten years of age is called Panner's disease. Because the prognosis for osteochondrosis of the capitellum is so much better when the patients are very young, Panner's disease is truly a distinct entity and worthy of its own name.

The proximal radioulnar joint is the articulation between the radial head and the radial notch (lesser sigmoid notch) of the ulna. The radioulnar joint allows for rotation of the radial head. This joint is rarely the cause of elbow symptoms in throwers.

CLINICAL PRESENTATION

Patients often present to clinicians with an insidious onset of elbow pain that gradually worsens with activity. Patients typically have pain while bending or straightening the elbow.

Mechanical symptoms may be present (popping/locking) and may indicate more advanced disease (loose body formation). The subjective complaint of stiffness is commonly reported.

Physical examination typically demonstrates a decreased range of motion when compared to the unaffected, contralateral extremity.

There may be a palpable effusion, crepitus, and tenderness to palpation. The location of tenderness may be sufficiently specific to point to the diagnosis. Pain at the radial head points to a diagnosis of osteochondritis dissecans of the capitellum. Pain and tenderness at the posteromedial tip of the olecranon will suggest valgus extension overload.

When palpating the soft tissues, the flexor-pronator muscles and the MCL are the most important structures to be examined. Pain among flexor-pronator masses indicates potential medial epicondylitis from an overload of stress and subtle instability of the elbow. Generally, medial epicondylitis caused by throwing strongly suggests MCL ligament damage. Pain or instability with valgus stress suggests a sprain of the ulnar collateral ligament.

OBJECTIVE EVIDENCE

All patients with persistent elbow pain should obtain plain radiographs of the elbow in full extension, and at 90 degrees of flexion (Figure 4).

Figure 4: AP radiograph showing a capitellar chondral lesion. (Image courtesy https://www.researchgate.net/figure/A-14-year-old-male-baseball-player-with-a-large-capitellar-osteochondritis-dissecans_fig4_321851321)

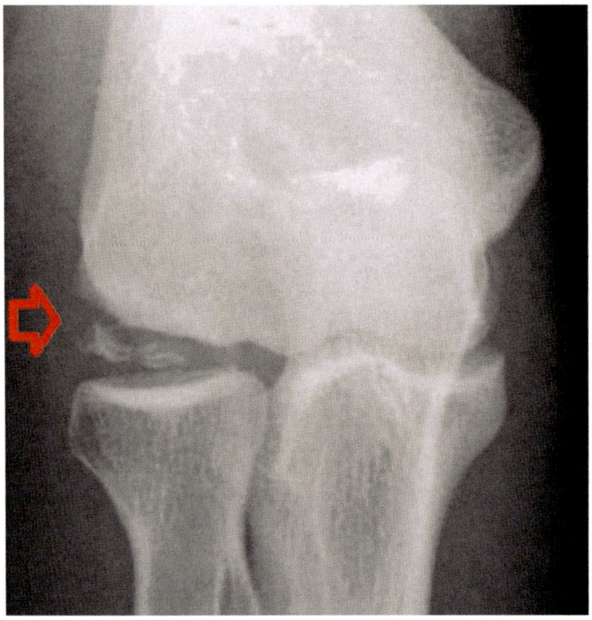

Magnetic resonance imaging is a valuable diagnostic tool in evaluating the articular surface as well as the ligaments nearby (Figure 5). These images should be scrutinized to determine if there is cartilage damage, bony collapse or loose fragments.

Figure 5: Coronal and sagittal MRI views of the elbow showing a displaced osteochondral fracture of the posterior capitellum (arrow) with associated marrow edema (asterisks). (Courtesy http://radsource.us/osteochondral-injury-of-the-elbow/)

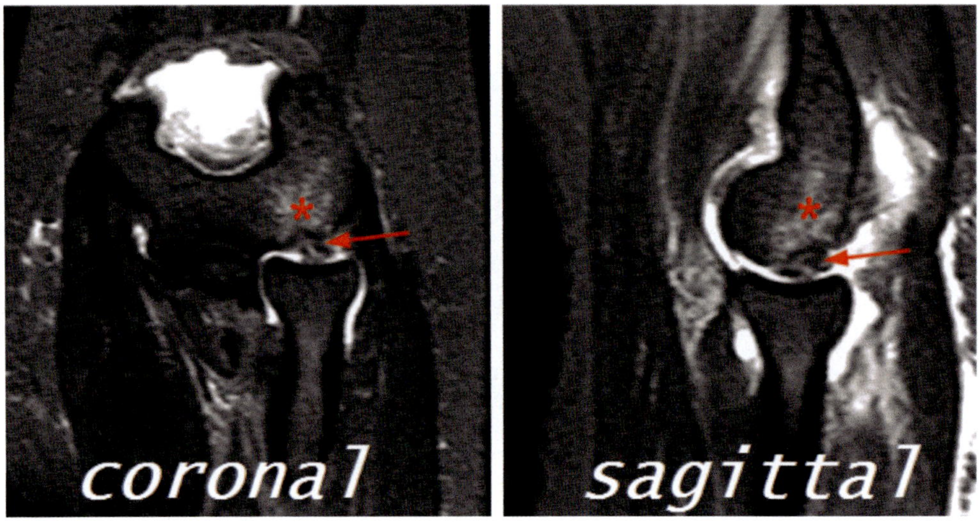

EPIDEMIOLOGY

Elbow pain is commonly seen in overhead throwing and non-throwing athletes, such as baseball pitchers, quarterbacks, volleyball and tennis players and gymnasts. The incidence of definitively diagnosed cartilage lesions (arthrosis) is low, but that may represent under-diagnosis.

The elbow is the second most common location for osteochondritis dissecans. (Note that the elbow is a distant second: a vast majority of osteochondritis dissecans lesions are found in the medial femoral condyle of the knee.)

Panner's disease is more commonly seen in males, however that may be a function of social forces – namely that males are more likely to participate in throwing sports.

DIFFERENTIAL DIAGNOSIS

Throwing, especially frequent throwing at high velocity, can exceed the capacity of the human body, and thus elbow pain is not uncommon in those who throw frequently at high velocity.

The differential diagnosis of elbow pain in throwing athletes includes tendonitis of the flexor/pronator tendons, sprains of the ulnar collateral ligament, irritation of the ulnar nerve, as well as articular surface pathologies described here. Stress fractures around growth plates may also produce the presenting symptoms.

RED FLAGS

There are no noteworthy red flag conditions.

TREATMENT OPTIONS AND OUTCOMES

The first-line treatment of elbow pain in throwing athletes is rest. A short course of immobilization may help reinforce the recommendation for rest. After approximately 3-6 weeks of rest, patients can gradually return to normal activities over the next 1-2 months. Non-steroidal anti-inflammatory medication (NSAID) can be administered for pain management.

Operative treatment is indicated for skeletally mature patients with symptomatic, unstable lesions or lesions that have failed to heal with the use of non-operative management.

Arthroscopic micro-fracture or drilling of the capitellum with or without loose body removal has been used as a surgical treatment of osteochondritis dissecans of the elbow. In this procedure, the surgeon penetrates the subchondral bone to allow blood to reach the affected area. The bleeding stimulates the growth of fibrocartilage to fill the lesion. Cartilage transfer procedures (popularly known by its acronym, OATS, standing for "osteochondral autograft transfer system") are another option. In this procedure, plugs of cartilage and bone are taken from a healthy area and are implanted to fill the lesion.

Fixation of the lesion is another surgical option which is indicated for larger lesions that are partially displaced or hinged.

Arthroscopic debridement and loose body excision is utilized for patients with unstable lesions who have catching or locking symptoms of the elbow.

Panner's disease is typically a self-limited condition that resolves once the epiphysis revascularizes and heals.

Outcomes are usually good in patients as long as there are no loose bodies; the presence of such bodies suggests more advanced disease. Recurrence of loose body formation and progression to arthritis is not uncommon.

Potential complications of treatment include elbow stiffness (especially from prolonged immobilization) and iatrogenic injury at surgery. Injury to the superficial radial, ulnar, posterior interosseous, medial antebrachial cutaneous, and anterior interosseous nerves can occur even with excellent technique. Infection is rare but possible.

RISK FACTORS AND PREVENTION

The primary risk factor for developing osteochondral lesions in the elbow is overuse, especially with activities that place significant compressive forces across the elbow. Too much throwing is harmful; pitch count limits should be observed especially in young players. Learning proper mechanics may also help reduce injury. It is critical that athletes do not continue to throw in the presence of symptoms.

MISCELLANY

The term "little leaguer's elbow" refers to any medial elbow injury in young throwing athletes, and may include medial epicondyle stress fractures, ulnar collateral ligament sprains or injuries to the flexor-pronator muscles.

KEY TERMS

Osteochondritis dissecans, Panner's disease, osteonecrosis, loose bodies, ulnohumeral articulation, radiocapitellar joint, proximal radioulnar joint, trochlea, capitellum

CHAPTER 14.

EPICONDYLITIS OF THE ELBOW

DESCRIPTION

Epicondylitis of the elbow is a misnomer because it is neither primarily a disease of the epicondyle, nor is it exclusively inflammatory (as the suffix "itis" would suggest).

Instead, epicondylitis is a condition of degenerative tendinopathy within the wrist extensor tendon (as in lateral epicondylitis) or flexor tendon (as in medial epicondylitis), tendons which originate at the elbow.

The common term "tennis elbow" refers to lateral epicondylitis which affects the origin of the wrist extensor muscles, while the term "golfer's elbow" refers to medial epicondylitis which affects the origin of the flexor/pronator muscles.

Epicondylitis is an overuse injury in which the rate of tendon damage exceeds the rate of tendon repair. This disequilibrium causes pain at the elbow and, ultimately, leads to impaired function – primarily in tasks that involve a power grip and require a stable wrist joint.

Figure 1: Surface landmark of the lateral epicondyle and the point of origin of the wrist extensor muscles.

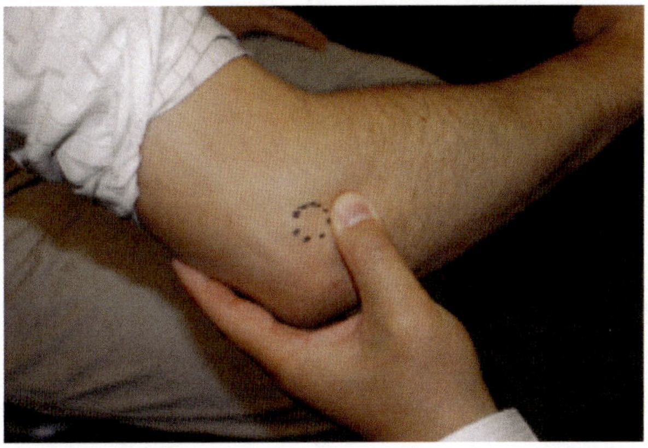

STRUCTURE AND FUNCTION

Epicondylitis is an overuse injury of the wrist extensor and flexor tendons including the extensor carpi radialis brevis, flexor carpi radialis, and pronator teres.

These muscles originate from the humerus (Figure 1) and cross the elbow joint, but their main action is at the wrist. They act at the wrist via concentric contraction (that is, shortening and changing the position of the joint), but they are also important in stabilizing the hand, wrist, and fingers, either isometrically (not moving at all) or via an eccentric contraction (actually lengthening while offering a resisting force). It is these eccentric contractions, defined as muscle contraction in one direction while another force elongates the muscle in the opposite direction, that are likely to cause microscopic tears within the tendon itself and its origin.

Lateral epicondylitis is commonly called "tennis elbow" because it is a common injury sustained by in tennis players hitting an off-center single arm backhand. When hitting the ball, the player's wrist extensors are active, to hold the wrist in position. When the tennis ball hits the racket, it applies a force on the wrist in the direction of flexion. This force pulls on the contracting extensor muscles and can create microscopic tears in the fibers that originate from the lateral epicondyle.

On the lateral side the primary focus of damage is within the extensor carpi radialis brevis; on the medial side it is within the flexor carpi radialis and pronator teres origin.

The histology of epicondylitis has been described as "angiofibroblastic hyperplasia": namely, the presence of fibroblasts and vascular tissue, along with degenerative and torn tendon fibers. (Note that pathological specimens are obtained at the time of surgery, and surgery is, of course, reserved for only severe cases. Thus, as far as we know, "angiofibroblastic hyperplasia" may be present only in end-stage disease.)

PATIENT PRESENTATION

Patients with epicondylitis present with a chief complaint of pain in the elbow on the affected side, especially with grasping.

Patients with epicondylitis often volunteer a history of repetitive forearm use, including sports involving rackets or bats, but also occupational activities such as working with tools.

In early phases of the condition, patients experience a minor ache after extensive activity. As the disease progresses, the signs and symptoms of epicondylitis are not only more severe, but may also be present without recent activity.

The presence of focal epicondylar pain and tenderness that is worse with provocation (stress on the wrist) is key to the physical diagnosis of epicondylitis.

Patients with epicondylitis complain of pain localized to the elbow; however, the best physical examination maneuver to provoke pain involves manipulation of the wrist, as the affected muscles are primarily used to stabilize the wrist. This is because while the lateral structures (especially the extensor carpi radialis brevis) are active wrist extensors, they also stabilize the wrist by resisting wrist flexion (with so-called eccentric or isometric contraction).

The importance of a stabilizing force against wrist flexion is seen dramatically in the mechanics of a tennis backhand stroke. This action requires that the wrist be held, fixed, in a neutral position despite the impulse of the ball, which, unopposed, would flex the wrist. A similar stabilizing force is employed on a routine basis in everyday grasping. Recall that the muscles of finger flexion originate on the volar surface of the forearm and cross the wrist on their journey to the phalanges. Unless these muscles are opposed by a countervailing wrist extension force, their firing will flex the wrist as well as the fingers. Put simply, in order to flex the fingers without flexing the wrist, the wrist extensor muscles must act. Repetitive grasping with the fingers therefore requires repetitive use of the wrist extensors, even if no wrist movement is produced.

Lateral epicondylitis can be caused by routine grasping tasks because they require the use of wrist extensors.

Symptoms of epicondylitis can be provoked on physical exam by asking the patient to hold his or her hand in maximal wrist extension, with the examiner acting against the patient to flex the wrist (Figure 2). Pain at the origin of the extensor muscles in the vicinity of the epicondyle is diagnostic. Note that the point of maximal tenderness is not at the epicondyle but is, rather, slightly distal, within the tendon itself.

Figure 2: Provocative examination of lateral epicondylitis. The patient is asked to actively extend the wrist against resistance; pain and tenderness near the origin of the wrist extensor muscles is a positive response.

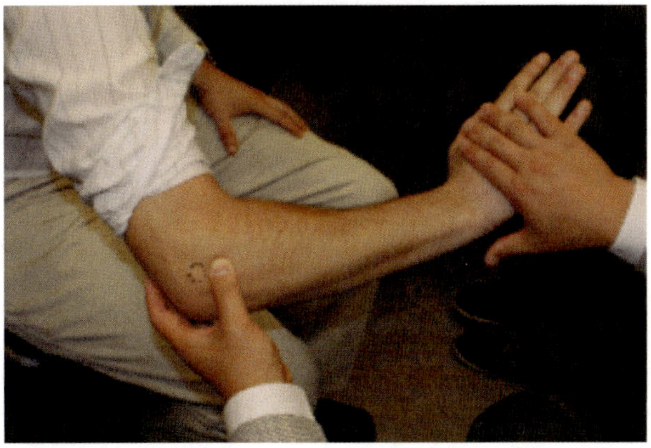

OBJECTIVE EVIDENCE

Epicondylitis is, for the most part, a clinical diagnosis: tenderness, especially provocative tenderness, in a patient with an apt history, makes the diagnosis.

An MRI (Figure 3) may show abnormal signal within the tendon at its origin, typically signifying chronic granulation tissue at the injured site. This test may also be used to exclude other conditions.

Figure 3: Elbow MRI with lateral epicondylitis (from radiopaedia.org http://bit.ly/1KSCmut)

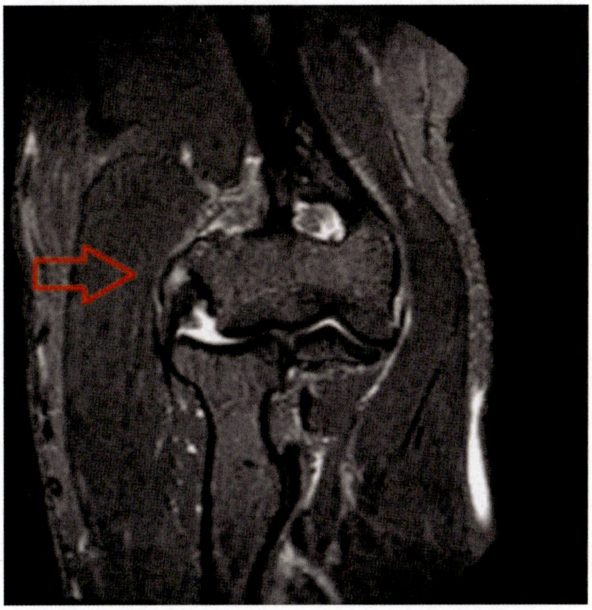

Similarly, an EMG may be helpful to exclude compression neuropathy. This is not 100% reliable, however. Plain radiographs may help exclude arthritis or loose bodies.

EPIDEMIOLOGY

The exact incidence of epicondylitis is not known, as there are mild forms of the condition that do not present for medical attention.

In general, it is safe to assume that epicondylitis is very common and should be high on the differential diagnosis of elbow pain.

Clinical experience suggests that medial epicondylitis is far less common than lateral epicondylitis. Moreover, the medial side of the elbow has other structures that may be the source of pain, e.g. the medial collateral ligament and the ulnar nerve. Medial epicondylitis therefore perhaps deserves a less prominent place on the "default" list of causes of medial elbow pain.

The incidence of epicondylitis is highest in the fourth and fifth decades of life. It can be present in both older and younger patients, but like most tendinopathies, epicondylitis is mostly prevalent in middle age.

DIFFERENTIAL DIAGNOSIS

Cubital tunnel syndrome, i.e., a compression neuropathy of the ulnar nerve at the elbow, is commonly seen in association with medial epicondylitis, but also may be seen on its own.

Entrapment of the radial nerve in the arcade of Frohse may mimic lateral epicondylitis (this can be diagnosed by EMG, clinical examination for radial tunnel syndrome, or diagnostic injection).

Cervical radiculopathy can also present as elbow pain: C5 or C6 nerve roots for lateral elbow pain; C8 or T1 nerve roots for medial elbow pain.

In addition, primary pathology within the joints, including arthritis, loose bodies and synovitis, may mimic the symptoms.

RED FLAGS

None

TREATMENT OPTIONS AND OUTCOMES

As epicondylitis is an overuse injury, it is best treated initially by a period of relative rest. Avoiding provocative activities, assuming they can be identified and omitted, may be helpful.

So-called "counterforce bracing" may also be helpful. This bracing involves a strap worn distal to the elbow that helps redirect force away from the origin (please see "Miscellany", below).

Splinting the wrist may also be helpful for this elbow pain (Figure 4). Note that the finger flexor tendons of course cross the wrist as well. As such, active finger flexion will flex the wrist unless there is a so-called isometric contraction of the wrist extensors. That is, wrist extension is needed to oppose the flexion force. By stabilizing the wrist with a brace, the wrist extensor muscles can rest even while grasping.

Figure 4: A wrist splint that may ameliorate elbow pain. By holding the wrist in a stable, fixed position, the brace allows the extensor muscles to rest during grasping. (From Flickr http://bit.ly/1PaqK82)

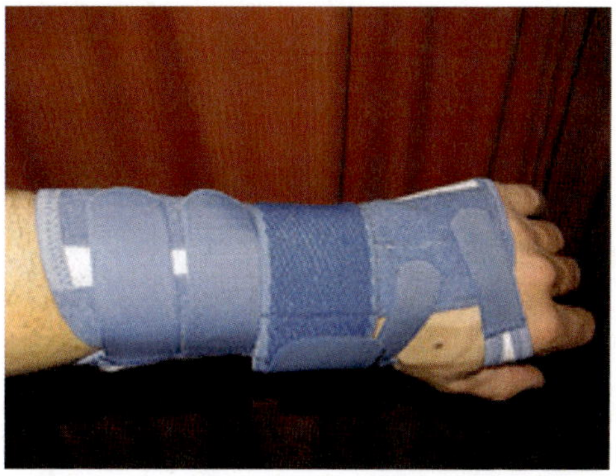

Physical therapy, especially modalities such as ultrasound and tendon glides, may be helpful.

Cortisone injections are also an accepted mode of treatment. Cortisone's precise mechanism of action is not known with certainty, however, it is relatively effective at minimizing pain in the short term.

Surgical treatment of epicondylitis is reserved for severe cases. Lateral epicondylitis can be treated by excision of the chronic granulation tissue of the extensor carpi radialis brevis and subsequent repair with appropriate immobilization while the tendon heals.

In general, patients with epicondylitis do well – especially if they interpret the pain as a signal to stop doing what is causing the pain. Pain, to the extent that it enforces a period of rest, promotes recuperation.

Controlled studies documenting the natural history of treated and untreated epicondylitis, however, have not been performed.

RISK FACTORS

Epicondylitis is an overuse injury that often occurs in the setting of aging. There is not much that can be done to prevent aging, of course. Patients who are entering the fourth and fifth decade of life, however, may need to modulate their activities accordingly.

It is also worth noting that poor form and technique – and the use of poorly maintained or adjusted equipment – may increase the risk of epicondylitis. For example, playing tennis with a racket poorly matched to one's skill and size may help inflict damage.

MISCELLANY

The concept of counterforce bracing (Figures 5 and 6) is similar to the capo used in a guitar, which effectively changes the "origin point" of the guitar string.

Figure 5: Counterforce bracing for epicondylitis

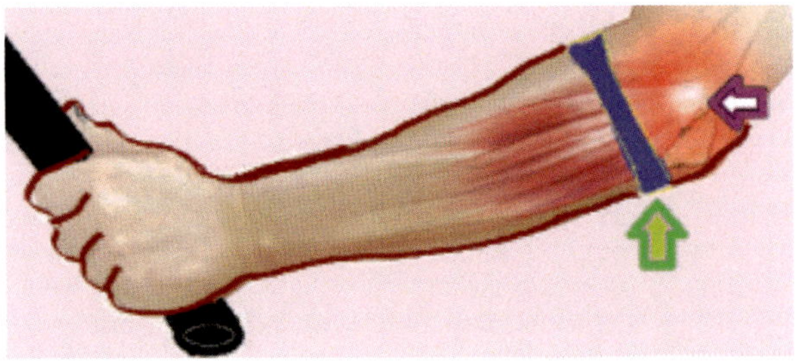

Figure 6: The guitar capo shown in the photo (Source: Flickr http://bit.ly/1nZsni5) effectively shortens the guitar strings, just as a strap on the forearm shortens the extensor muscles. This shortening creates a new virtual point of origin (shown by the green arrow in Figure 5) and shields the proximal origin of the extensor tendons (purple arrow) and thereby allows it to rest and recover.

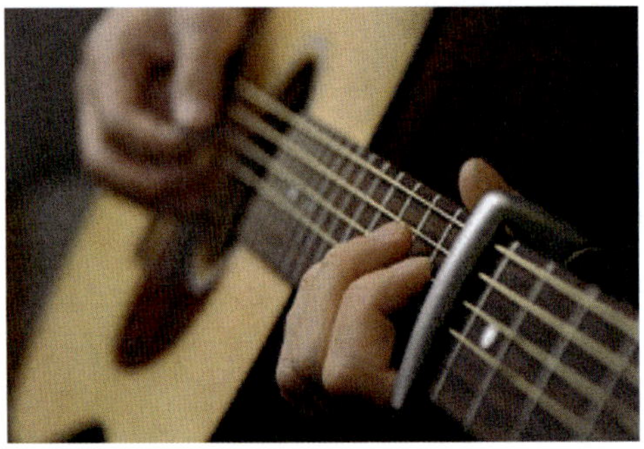

Just as a dog can have lice and fleas, a patient can have two simultaneous conditions, e.g. lateral and medial epicondylitis. This combination of tennis and golfer's elbow has been described by Nirschl as "country club elbow."

KEY TERMS

Epicondylitis, angiofibroblastic hyperplasia

SKILLS AND COMPETENCIES

Perform physical examination to diagnose epicondylitis.

CHAPTER 15.

TENDON DISORDERS OF THE HIP AND THIGH

DESCRIPTION

The hip is surrounded by powerful muscles; disorders of these muscles and their associated tendons and bursas are frequently seen in athletes. The muscles usually affected include the hamstrings posteriorly; the adductor muscles of the medial thigh; the muscles that cross the anterior aspect of the hip and flex it, notably, the iliopsoas; and on the lateral side, the gluteus medius and minimus (with its associated trochanteric bursa) and tensor fascia lata (and its broad expansion into the iliotibial band). These muscles are important not only for moving the hip but also for stabilizing the pelvis, and thus, once injured, can produce symptoms even with minimal activity. Happily, most disorders of the muscles, tendons and bursas around the hip are self-limited and resolve with rest and other mild treatments.

In this section, the following tendon-related disorders will be considered:

- Hamstring injury,
- Adductor strain,
- Snapping hip syndrome,
- Greater trochanteric pain syndrome,
- Iliotibial band syndrome.

HAMSTRING INJURY

The hamstrings (Figure 1) comprise three muscles, originating, for the most part, from the ischial tuberosity. (The exception is the short head of the biceps, which originates from the posterior aspect of the proximal femur.) Two of the hamstrings are medial, the semitendinosus and semimembranosus, and insert on the tibia; the biceps femoris is lateral and inserts on the fibula. The hamstrings extend the hip and flex the knee. They also a have small rotatory effect on the lower leg. The hamstrings also decelerate knee extension and assist the anterior cruciate ligament to help prevent anterior tibial subluxation.

Figure 1: The hamstrings: the semimembranosus (blue line), semitendinosus (black line) and biceps femoris (orange line). (Modified from https://en.wikipedia.org/wiki/Hamstring#/media/File:Pulled_Hamstring.png)

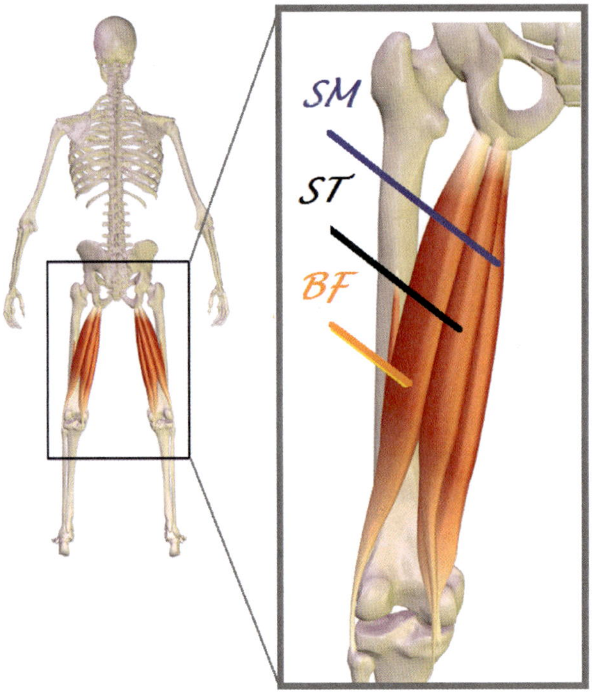

Injuries of the hamstring range from strains of the muscle (also known as a "pulled hamstring") to complete tears within the muscle or avulsion of the tendon from its origin on the ischium.

The hamstring muscle-tendon unit is injured when it is exposed to forces beyond the tolerance of the tissue. Often this force is applied during so-called "eccentric contraction". The term "eccentric" acknowledges that the muscle is actually being elongated, despite its attempt to "contract". (Weightlifters call this "negative work.") Eccentric contraction of the hamstrings is seen during running. With each step, the quadriceps swings the leg forward, by flexing the hip and extending the knee. This motion passively stretches the hamstrings. Yet as the leg swings forward, the hamstrings contract eccentrically to decelerate the hip flexion and knee extension. Indeed, the greatest force is applied when the hamstrings are at their maximal length. At this point, the muscle-tendon unit is particularly susceptible to injury.

The hamstrings are the most commonly injured hip/thigh muscle group. People with less flexibility or excessively strong quadriceps muscles (creating imbalance) are more vulnerable to injury.

Acute hamstring injuries are characterized by a sudden, sharp pain in the thigh, with swelling and/or ecchymosis (bluish discoloration of the skin from extravasation of blood) appearing over the next few hours (Figure 2).

Figure 2: Clinical photograph, 4 days after a left hamstring injury.

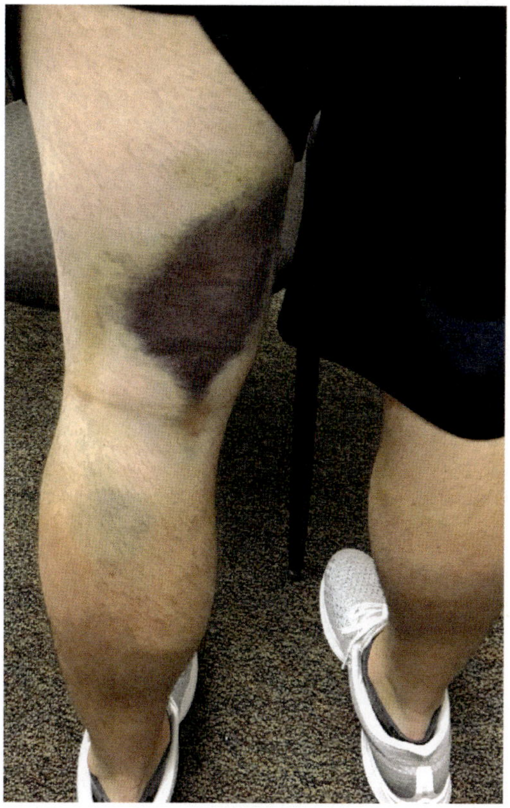

Because of pain or actual tissue failure, there will be weakness that may cause the injured athlete to fall or stumble when the injury is sustained.

The mainstay of the physical examination is tenderness over the affected area, with a characteristic short arc gait (to minimize tension on the hamstrings). If there is a myotendinous rupture, a mass may be palpable in the middle third of the posterior thigh.

X-rays may be obtained routinely, but are specifically indicated if there is a suspected tendon avulsion. Magnetic Resonance Imaging may be helpful to determine the extent of the injury.

Most hamstring strains heal with rest, followed by a course of physical therapy to restore range of motion and strength. Surgery is reserved for bony avulsion injuries or large tears when the tendon has retracted more than 2 cm.

Note that lumbar spondylolisthesis (in which a vertebra slips forward relative to an adjacent one) could present with hamstring pain and tightness.

ADDUCTOR STRAIN

There are three named adductor muscles (adductor longus, adductor magnus and adductor brevis) and three other muscles (gracilis, obturator externus and pectineus) that adduct the hip. Of these, the adductor longus (Figure 3) is the most commonly injured muscle.

Figure 3: The adductor longus. (courtesy of https://www.hindawi.com/journals/crior/2015/840540/fig1/)

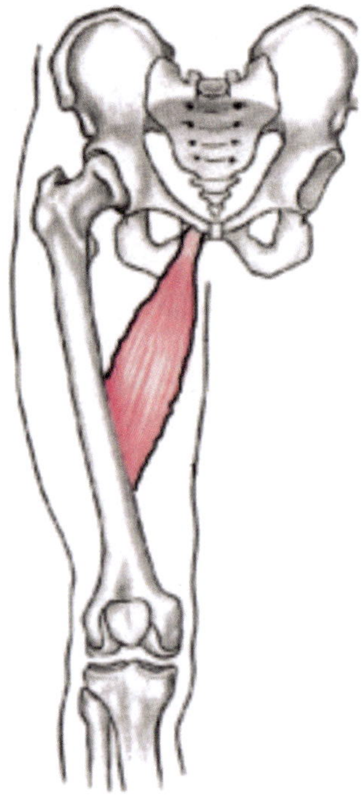

Strains of the adductor muscle group, also known as a "pulled groin," are caused by forceful abduction or external rotation of the leg while the adductors are firing (as may be seen when kicking or swinging the leg, and colliding with another player or stationary object). Strains of the adductor muscle group are more commonly seen in soccer and hockey players where this type of motion is more frequently encountered. The adductor muscle group is the second most commonly injured muscle group.

Patients with adductor strains present with immediate and severe groin pain, with tenderness often extending above and below the site of injury. There will be pain with passive abduction, and decreased strength on adduction compared to the other leg.

In general, strains of the adductor muscle are acute events. Sub-acute or chronic complaints may suggest a non-musculoskeletal cause for the groin pain including hernias and disorders of the urogenital system.

AP pelvis x-rays may show a fleck of bone, but in general, imaging is used not so much to confirm this diagnosis, but to rule out other causes of groin pain such as osteitis pubis, avulsion fractures or stress fractures.

Rest, followed by a course of physical therapy to restore range of motion and strength, is the preferred treatment; there are no indications for surgery. Unfortunately, groin strains may recur; patients should be counseled against returning to sports too quickly and encouraged to warm up and stretch adequately before activities.

GREATER TROCHANTERIC PAIN SYNDROME

The gluteus medius and minimus originate in the ileum and insert on the greater trochanter of the femur. Their primary function is hip abduction, notably resisting hip adduction when standing on one leg. (When standing on one leg, the body's center of gravity is medial to the hip joint, such that without resistance, the hip joint would passively adduct, causing the pelvis to tilt. Isometric hip abduction force by the glutei keep the pelvis level. Indeed, dysfunction of the glutei is the basis of so-called Trendelenburg gait, in which a patient lurches to the weakened side to maintain a level pelvis, on average, throughout the gait cycle.)

Tendinopathy of the gluteus medius and minimus, along with inflammation of the bursa near their insertion on the trochanter, is a common source of lateral hip pain (Figure 4).

Figure 4: The classic location of greater trochanteric pain. (courtesy of https://www.physio-pedia.com/Gluteal_Tendinopathy)

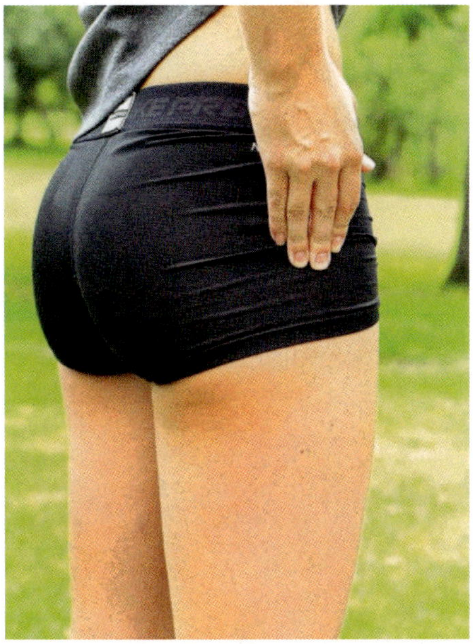

Because tendinopathy and bursitis coexist, the term "greater trochanteric pain syndrome" may be preferable.

Among people age 50 to 70 years, greater trochanteric pain syndrome is found in ~15% of females and ~5% of males.

The most common examination finding is tenderness to palpation of the greater trochanter; there is no objective criterion for the diagnosis.

The treatment of greater trochanteric pain syndrome is non-operative. Pain relief medication (including NSAIDs, on the assumption that chronic tendinopathy contributes to the symptoms) along with physical therapy and corticosteroid injection have been used. Yet because many patients will have resolution of their symptoms even without treatment, it is unclear what is most effective. Conditions that do not resolve may be treated with low-energy extracorporeal shock wave therapy. Platelet-rich plasma injections have been proposed to treat tendinopathies, however reliable evidence of efficacy is not yet in hand.

Trochanteric bursectomy with or without tendon lengthening may also be tried for patients who do not respond to non-operative management.

SNAPPING HIP SYNDROME

The iliopsoas is the confluence of psoas and the iliacus muscles. These have separate origins in the abdomen but attach as one on the lesser trochanter (Figure 5). It is the strongest flexor of the hip.

Figure 5: The course of the iliopsoas over the hip joint. (modified from https://en.wikipedia.org/wiki/Iliacus_muscle)

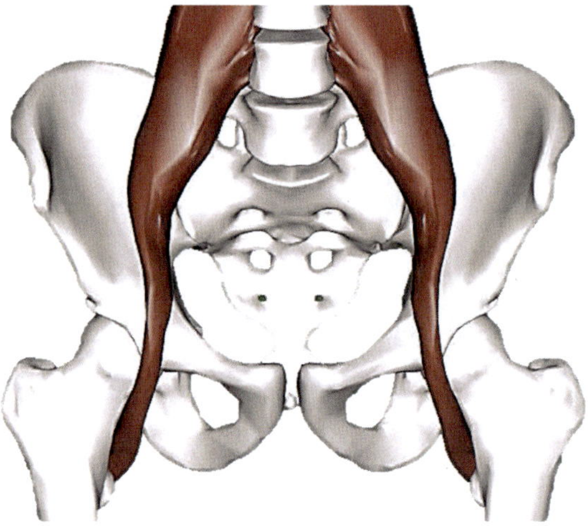

The tensor fascia lata originates from anterior superior iliac spine and attaches into the iliotibial band in the upper thigh. The iliotibial band then inserts on Gerdy's tubercle on the proximal lateral tibia (Figure 6).

Figure 6: The course of the tensor fascia lata (TFL) and iliotibial band (ITB) on the lateral thigh. (modified from https://www.physio-pedia.com/File:Itbs.png)

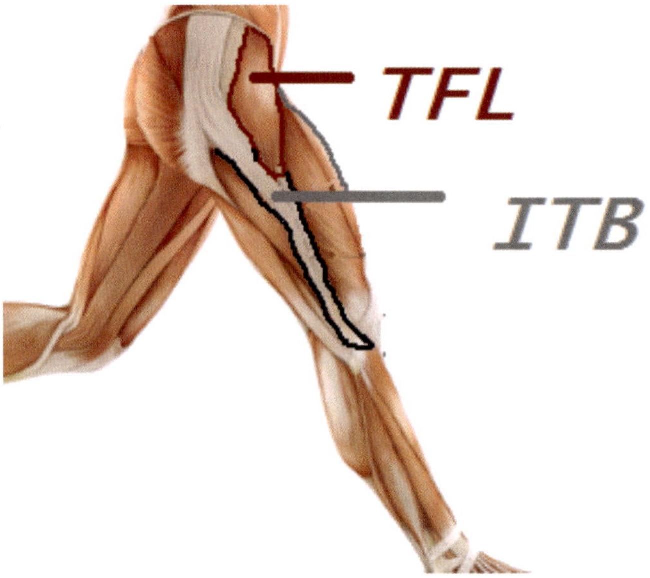

The tensor fasciae lata can actively move the hip and knee joints, but its main function is to resist the forces of other muscles and thereby stabilize the lower extremity during gait.

Snapping hip syndrome is the term applied to the snapping sensation a patient may perceive when the hip is flexed and extended. This sensation may be perceived via either a sound or mechanical pop.

The snap usually has an extra-articular (muscular) cause. When the sensation is perceived laterally, snapping hip syndrome is caused by the tensor fasciae lata, or gluteus medius tendon sliding across the greater trochanter of the femur. When the snapping is medial, the cause is likely to be the iliopsoas tendon catching on a process of the pelvis or the lesser trochanter of the femur.

Snapping hip syndrome of an extra-articular cause is usually painless, though friction may lead to a local bursitis.

Snapping of the hip could be due to intra-articular pathology, such as a labral tear. This version is more often symptomatic and the "snap" is more of a "click". Here, pain is more common.

Snapping hip is most common in athletes and dancers in their teens.

On exam, snapping of the hip due to the iliopsoas tendon sliding over the femoral head can be reproduced by passively extending and internally rotating the hip from a flexed and externally rotated position.

Dynamic ultrasound can demonstrate tendon subluxation. MRI can be used to identify intra-articular pathology. The "danger" of MRI is the detection of incidental intra-articular pathology, with the snapping indeed caused by the tendon (and not by other, incidental findings).

Painless snapping should be treated with reassurance only. Pain from bursitis may be treated with a short course of rest and stretching. Should that not work, injections may help. In the most refractory cases, surgical release of the contracted tissue may be indicated.

ILIOTIBIAL BAND SYNDROME

As noted, the tensor fascia lata originates from the pelvis but inserts in the tibia. It may be the source of distal thigh or knee pain accordingly. The function of the tensor fasciae lata at the knee is unusual in that depending on the position of the knee, it is either a flexor or extensor. If the knee is flexed already, the iliotibial band is behind the center of rotation and thus helps flex the knee even more, but in a position close to terminal knee extension, its line of pull is anterior and thus extends the knee. Because the iliotibial band contacts the distal lateral femur when the knee is in motion, it is subject to irritation and inflammation. This is termed iliotibial band syndrome.

Patients with iliotibial band syndrome present with activity-related lateral knee pain of insidious onset, localized to the contact point of the lateral femoral epicondyle and the iliotibial band as it courses distally to the knee. To confirm on physical exam, the patient is placed in a lateral decubitus position (affected side up) with the hip slightly flexed and the examiner passively flexes the knee. If pain is produced only with compression of the iliotibial band, this test is considered positive.

Because Iliotibial band syndrome may be present in 10-25% of runners, and is essentially not found among those who do not run, it is considered a classic overuse syndrome. The logical treatment is thus under-use, that is, relative rest.

Iliotibial band dysfunction is thought to be caused primarily by a "naturally" tight iliotibial band, but the observed association with excessive running in the same direction on an indoor (curved) track suggests that running on a gradient may be a cause too. The tight iliotibial band may be addressed with stretching exercises.

Lateral knee joint line tenderness, distal to the femur, suggests meniscal injury or arthritis rather than iliotibial band syndrome.

MISCELLANY

- Filet mignon is a beef steak cut of the psoas muscle.
- Genesis 32:32 refers to "the tendon attached to the socket of the hip" though no tendon literally attaches to the socket.
- Snapping hip is also known as coxa saltans. The word "saltans" refers to dancing or jumping. The former meaning is probably intended with the hip condition (as it is found in dancers); the latter meaning is seen with the medical term "saltatory conduction", that is the propagation of action potentials along myelinated axons jumping from one node of Ranvier to the next. It is also used in the named Italian dish, veal saltimbocca – food so good it is said to jump into your mouth.

KEY TERMS

adductor longus, biceps femoris, gluteus medius, greater trochanter, iliopsoas, iliotibial band, lesser trochanter, semimembranosus, semitendinosus, tensor fascia lata

SKILLS

Identify the hip muscle(s) responsible for symptoms. Demonstrate stretching exercises for tight hip muscles. Prepare veal saltimbocca for a party of 6, to be accompanied by a nice chianti.

CHAPTER 16.

LABRAL TEARS OF THE HIP AND FEMOROACETABULAR IMPINGEMENT

DESCRIPTION

The acetabular labrum is a rim of cartilage surrounding the socket of the hip joint. Damage to the labrum can result from various causes, including trauma and degeneration. Labral tears can be painful, but also may be found incidentally on imaging studies. Femoroacetabular impingement is a clinical syndrome associated with labral tears. This syndrome is characterized by bony overgrowth of either the femur, the pelvis or both (Figure 1). These morphological abnormalities are thought to produce (or at least reflect) abnormal contact between the proximal femur and acetabulum during hip flexion and rotation. It has been proposed that this contact damages the labrum as well as the articular cartilage of the hip joint itself.

Figure 1: Schematic tracing of the bones of the hip joint, showing the normal femur and pelvis in red. The bony overgrowth impingement is shown in black. (The green arrow points to so-called "cam impingement" and the blue arrow to "pincer impingement" [see text]).

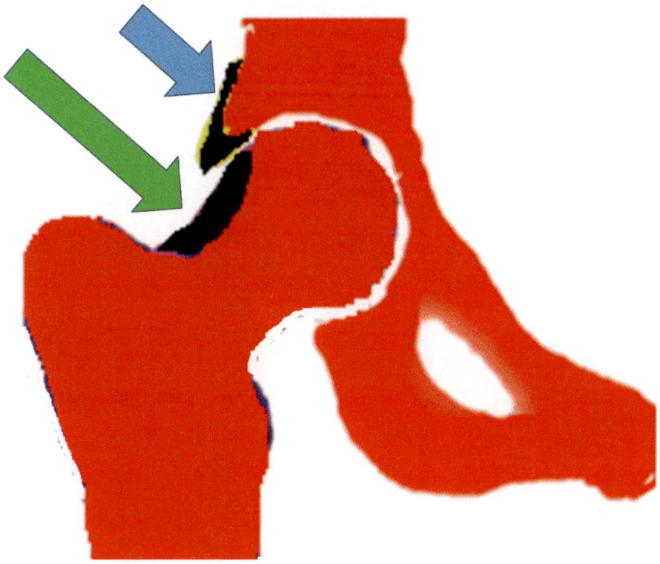

STRUCTURE AND FUNCTION

The labrum is a fibrocartilaginous structure surrounding the rim of the acetabulum (Figure 2). In cross section, the labrum is triangular with an articular and capsular surface. The labrum rim functions to deepen the acetabulum, increasing the contact area of the hip joint and thereby reducing cartilage contact pressure and increasing hip stability.

Figure 2: The labrum, outlined in red, serves to deepen the socket of the acetabulum.

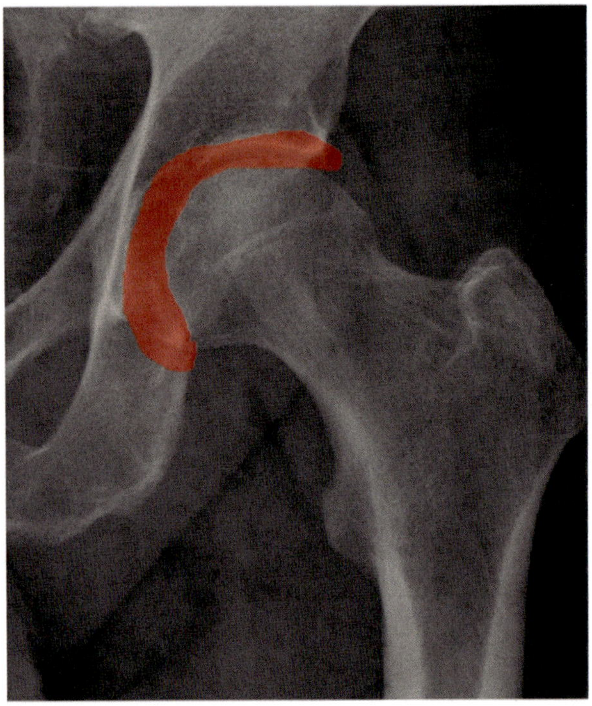

Trauma is a common cause of labral tears. Usually, this involves a mechanism which results in forceful resistance of hip flexion (e.g. tackled while kicking or running).

Hip dysplasia and capsular laxity are associated with labral tears, likely by exposing the labrum to abnormal forces.

Femoroacetabular impingement anatomy is also associated with labral tears. It is important to distinguish between "femoroacetabular impingement anatomy" –that is, the anatomic morphological deviance from normal– and the clinical syndrome of femoroacetabular impingement, which is the combination of the characteristic anatomy and clinical symptoms. Many people have femoroacetabular impingement anatomy without symptoms.

Femoroacetabular impingement anatomy is broadly defined by bony overgrowth of the femur at the femoral head-neck junction, termed "Cam impingement" (Figure 3), or overgrowth of the acetabular rim, termed "Pincer impingement" (Figure 4). Both Cam and Pincer impingement may be found concurrently.

Figures 3a: An x-ray of cam impingement.

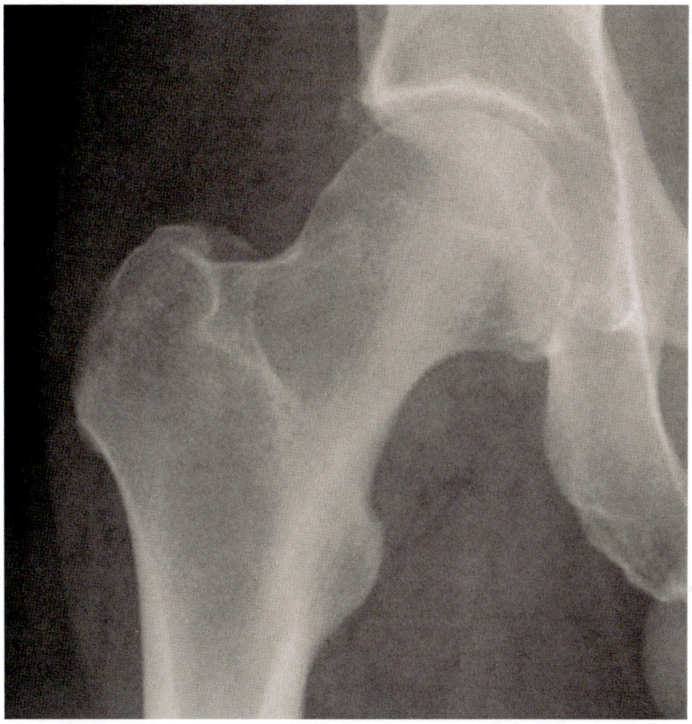

In Figure 3b, the x-ray of Figure 3 is annotated. The normal contour of the femur shown in Figure 3a is shaded in purple. The red arrow points to the excess bone causing cam impingement. (Case courtesy of Dr. Kenny Sim, Radiopaedia.org, rID: 30914)

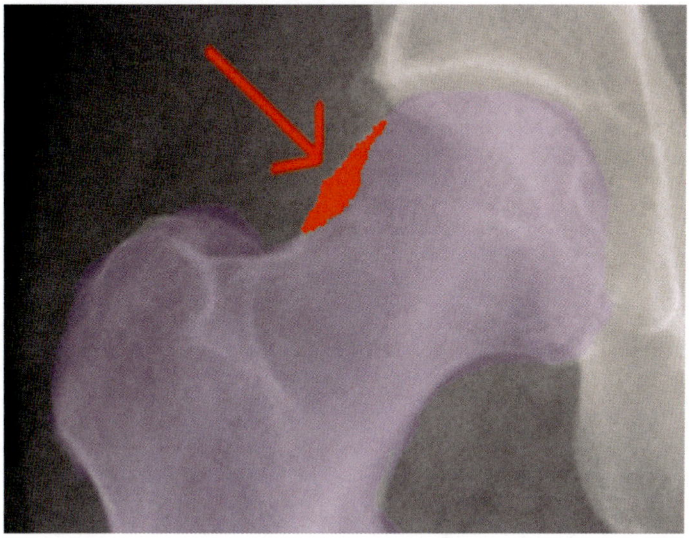

Figure 4: Pincer impingement. The outline of a normal pelvis is shaded in red. The yellow arrow points to the excess acetabular bone seen in pincer impingement. (Case courtesy of A.Prof Frank Gaillard, Radiopaedia.org, rID: 2738)

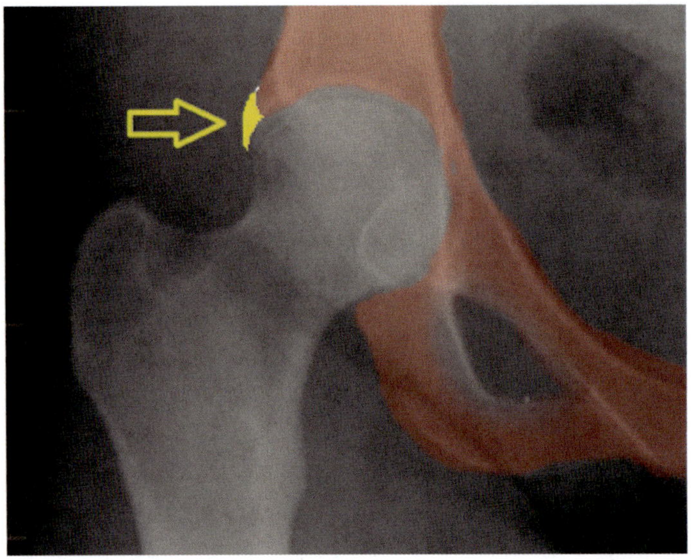

Cam impingement is characterized by a non-spherical femoral head and decreased head-neck offset. During hip flexion, the aspherical femoral head can make contact that shears the acetabular cartilage and the labrum. Labral damage in Cam deformity most often occurs anterosuperiorly, at the transition zone where the labrum blends into the hyaline cartilage.

Pincer impingement is due to acetabular overgrowth and "over-coverage" of the femur. Abnormal contact between the overgrown acetabular rim and femoral head-neck junction leads to tears within the substance of the labrum. Pincer-associated labral tears are also most often in the anterosuperior quadrant of the labrum, though a so-called contrecoup cartilage lesion in the posteroinferior acetabulum may be found as well.

PATIENT PRESENTATION

Patients with labral tears may present with hip pain and may note clicking, locking, and popping as well. In almost all patients, the pain is located in the anterior hip or groin.

Patients may make a "C sign" – grasping the affected hip with their hand indicating both anterior and posterior hip pain (Figure 5).

Figure 5: Demonstration of the "C sign." Patients with labral tears, when asked to "point" to the area of pain will not point but rather grasp the hip, as shown.

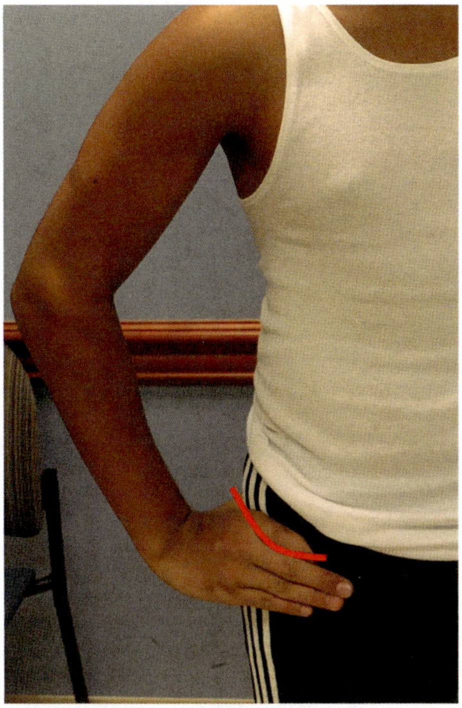

On physical exam, flexion, adduction, and internal rotation (Figure 6) can provoke the symptoms of an anterior-superior tear whereas abduction and external rotation (Figure 7) tend to elicit pain in those with posterior labral tears.

Figure 6: Patients with an anterior-superior labral tear will report pain if the examiner passively flexes (red arrow), slightly adducts (white arrow) and internally rotates (green arrow) the hip.

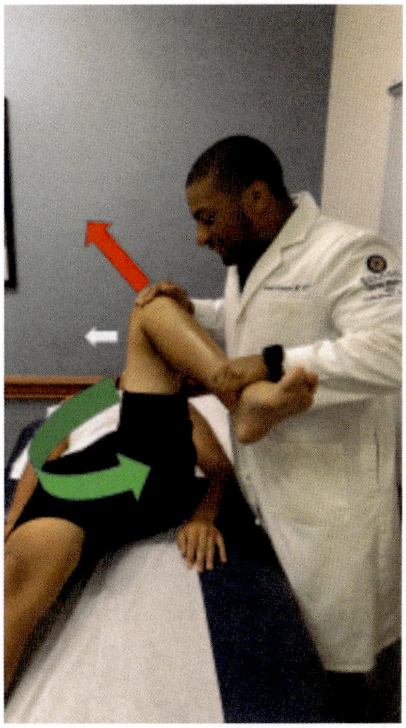

Figure 7: Patients with posterior labral tears will report pain if the examiner abducts (white arrow) and externally rotates (green arrow) the hip.

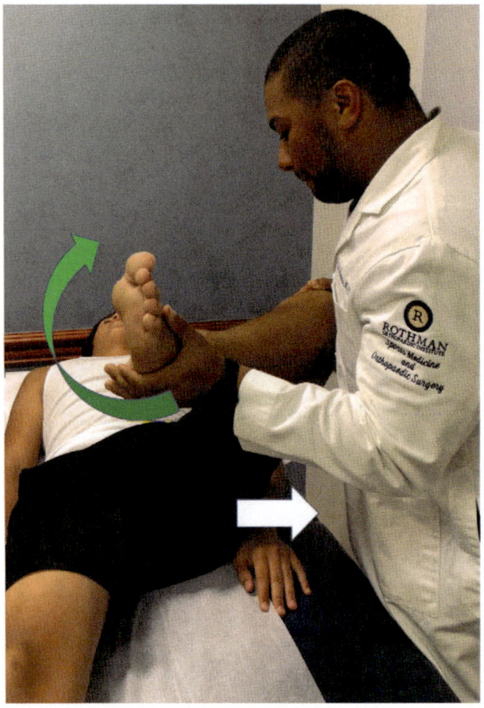

These tests are performed when the patient is supine and the hip and knee are flexed to 90 degrees.

Hip range of motion may be limited, especially in rotation, but this is not a specific finding.

OBJECTIVE EVIDENCE

MRI is the most sensitive method of imaging and study of choice to evaluate for chondral or labral damage (Figure 8).

Figure 8: A labral tear seen on hip MRI. (Case courtesy of Dr Roberto Schubert, Radiopaedia.org, rID: 13826)

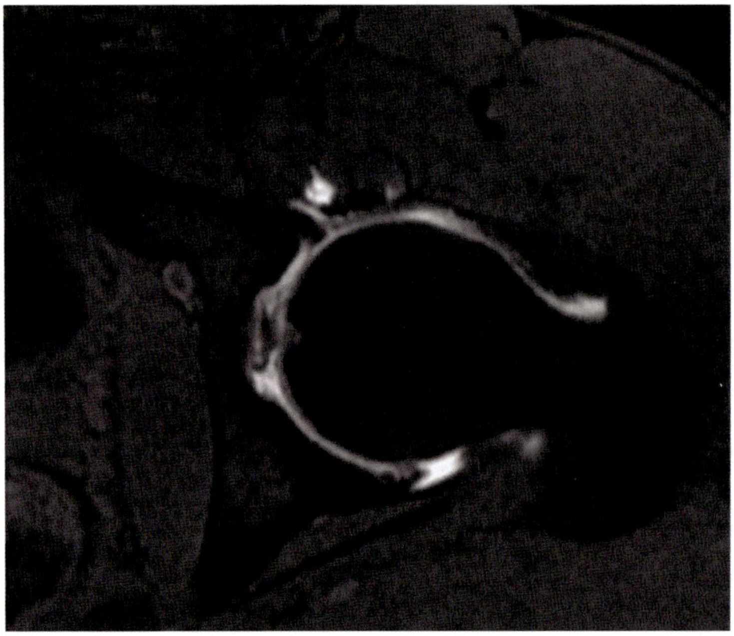

Nonetheless, MRI may miss clinically significant findings. MRI arthrogram (MRI with contrast material injected into the joint), is the study of choice to identify labral tears.

CT scans help better characterize the bony deformities in femoroacetabular impingement and assist in surgical planning.

Most patients with labral tears (85% or more) have some radiographic abnormality. That is to say, labral tears are rarely found in hips with normal bony anatomy. Thus, while normalcy does not exclude the diagnosis, it makes it less likely.

(Note that the finding that most patients with labral tears have some radiographic abnormality does not mean that these abnormalities *cause* the tear. For one thing, there may be many people with these abnormalities that do not have a tear. The other possibility is that the radiographic abnormality, e.g. bone overgrowth, is caused by the labral tear, and not the other way around.)

Initial radiographic evaluation of patients with symptoms concerning for femoroacetabular impingement or labral pathology should be an anterior posterior pelvis and lateral hip film. Frog leg or cross table lateral may also be used. However, a 45 degrees Dunn lateral (hip flexed to 45 degrees and abducted 20 degrees) provides the most revealing view of a potential femoroacetabular impingement deformity.

Multiple studies focusing on prevalence data in femoroacetabular impingement have shown that 24-50% of asymptomatic patients have radiographic signs of femoroacetabular impingement. These data highlight the importance of clinically correlating imaging when assessing a patient who might have femoroacetabular impingement.

In Cam impingement, alpha angle is a commonly used quantitative measure of the deformity. This angle is determined by placing a circle over the femoral head with a line from the center of the circle to the center of the femoral neck and another line from the center of the circle to the first point of the superior head-neck junction (Figures 9 and 10).

Figure 9: The alpha angle is formed by two lines emanating from the center of the femoral head: one bisecting the femoral neck and second drawn to the point where the neck meets the head. Normal anatomy is shown here.

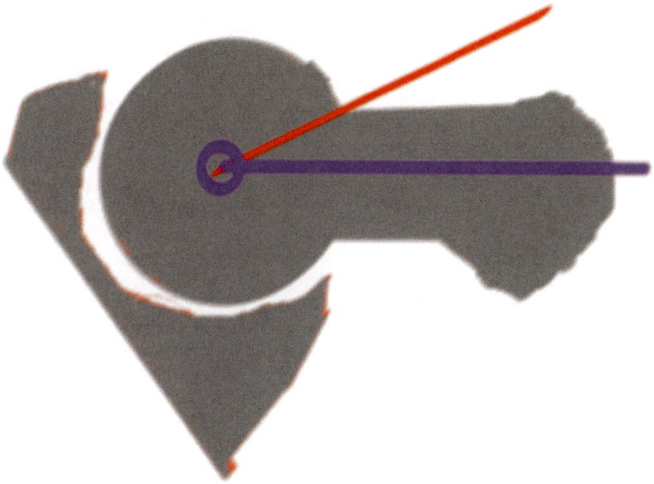

Figure 10: In this drawing, there is bony overgrowth from a cam lesion (green) which changes the point where the neck meets the head, leading to a larger alpha angle.

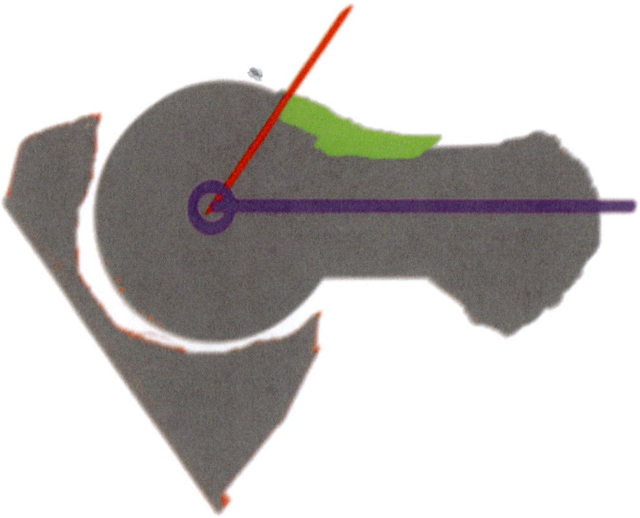

The higher the angle between these two lines, the larger and more severe the Cam lesion. However, there is no precise criterion value for alpha angle that defines pathological abnormality and (interestingly) the original paper in *Clinical Orthopaedics and Related Research* describing femoroacetabular impingement did not mention the alpha angle.

Alpha angles are most accurate when obtained from special MRI scans which control for hip rotation.

Radiographs in Pincer type impingement reveal acetabular over coverage on the AP pelvis plain film. There may also be retroversion of the femoral neck.

A classic finding of Pincer impingement due to acetabular retroversion is the crossover sign, in which the anterior rim of the acetabulum crosses the line of the posterior aspect of the rim prior to the lateral aspect of acetabulum

Center edge angle is another measurement used to assess for acetabular over coverage leading to Pincer type impingement.

EPIDEMIOLOGY

Labral tears have the highest incidence in patients with acetabular dysplasia.

Cam impingement anatomy is more commonly seen in young males. Pincer lesions are more frequently seen in middle-aged females.

The most common subtype of femoroacetabular impingement is combined, or a component of both Cam and Pincer impingement.

Needless to say, all anatomic measures, including the roundness of the proximal femur and amount of anterior acetabular coverage lie on a continuum, with no perfect criterion separating normal from abnormal. With a sufficiently lax definition, nearly all people have some degree of femoroacetabular impingement anatomy.

DIFFERENTIAL DIAGNOSIS

There are numerous pathologies that can lead to pain at the hip or groin. Extra-articular injury of muscles and tendons are the most common source of hip and groin pain in young active adults. Thus, one must consider muscle strains and tendinopathies.

Snapping hip may produce symptoms resembling mechanical hip pain seen in femoroacetabular impingement or labral tear. Bursitis, particularly iliopectineal bursitis, produces groin pain and increased pain with hip flexion.

Neuropathies should also be included in the differential for hip/groin pain. While obturator or ilioinguinal nerve entrapments may cause discomfort in the groin, these conditions often are associated with paresthesias or neurologic symptoms.

Stress fractures of the femoral neck and pubic rami must also be considered in patients presenting with hip/groin pain especially in thin long-distance runners.

Osteitis pubis (inflammation of the pubic symphysis) and groin muscle strains (also known as athletic pubalgia or "sports hernia") may cause hip pain similar to that of labral tears.

Hip osteoarthritis can cause groin pain, especially in older patients.

RED FLAGS

A stress fracture of the femoral neck may be the source of the presenting complaints and should not be missed. Pain that is related to activity and not changed by position of the hip joint should increase the suspicion of this diagnosis, especially in patients at risk for stress fractures.

TREATMENT OPTIONS AND OUTCOMES

Nonoperative treatment, centering on rest, anti-inflammatory pain medications and physical therapy, should be the initial treatment for most patients with labral tears. While no universal physical therapy regiment has been defined, plans of rehabilitation focusing on hip strength and mobility in conjunction with posture and core strength have intuitive appeal.

Intra-articular hip injections can be considered but their efficacy has not been proven. A lack of a response to a preoperative injection is predictive of poor short term surgical outcomes.

Operative treatment of labral tears can involve labral resection, re-fixation, or reconstruction of soft tissue. However, studies have shown labral re-fixation results in better outcomes and decreased cartilage degeneration in comparison to resection.

Because of the high prevalence of femoroacetabular impingement morphology in asymptomatic patients, it is speculative at best to suggest that any treatment should be employed in the name of altering the risk of arthritis later in life. It may be more reasonable to address femoroacetabular impingement bony deformities when surgery is undertaken to repair the labrum: osteoplasty of the Cam deformity or resection of the Pincer lesion may be chosen.

RISK FACTORS AND PREVENTION

Hip dysplasia is the most common cause/risk factor for developing a labral tear.

According to the classic report on femoroacetabular impingement, "patients with otherwise normal or near-normal anatomic structure of the hip [can] experience impingement as a result of subjecting the hip to excessive and supraphysiologic ROM."

A history of a slipped epiphysis can lead to femoral neck retroversion and place patients at a risk for Cam impingement. Likewise, acetabular protrusion and coxa profunda predispose patients to Pincer impingement.

KEY TERMS

Femoroacetabular impingement, cam lesion, pincer lesion, hip labrum

SKILLS

Perform physical examination to suggest or exclude the diagnosis of labral disease.

CHAPTER 17.

DISORDERS OF THE EXTENSOR MECHANISM OF THE KNEE

DESCRIPTION

The extensor mechanism of the knee comprises the quadriceps muscle and tendon, the patella, and the patellar tendon (also known as the infra-patellar ligament). Disruption of any of these components impedes a person's ability to actively extend the knee or resist passive flexion. Such injuries are therefore incompatible with normal walking and standing. Failure of the quadriceps or patellar tendon is often, but not always, preceded by painful tendinopathy.

STRUCTURE AND FUNCTION

The quadriceps muscle, as its name implies, is composed of four muscles: the vastus lateralis, vastus intermedius, vastus medialis and rectus femoris (see Figure 1). All but part of the rectus femoris originate on the femur itself. These muscles converge at a point approximately 5 cm proximal to the patella to form the quadriceps tendon. The quadriceps tendon has multiple layers, with the rectus femoris as the most superficial layer, the vastus medialis and lateralis as the middle layer, and the vastus intermedius as the deepest layer. The superficial layer is well vascularized; however, there is a hypovascular zone in the middle and deep layers approximately 1-2 cm proximal to the patella. This is the most common site of rupture.

The patellar tendon originates at the distal end of the anterior aspect of the patella and inserts on the anterior aspect of the tibia at the tibial tuberosity. The tendon most commonly tears at its origination on the patella.

Figure 1: Anatomy of the extensor mechanism. The quadriceps muscles are outlined in red, and their common tendon and the infrapatellar ligament are in yellow. Both attach to the patella, outlined in gray. (Original x-rays from https://radiopaedia.org/cases/normal-knees-x-rays)

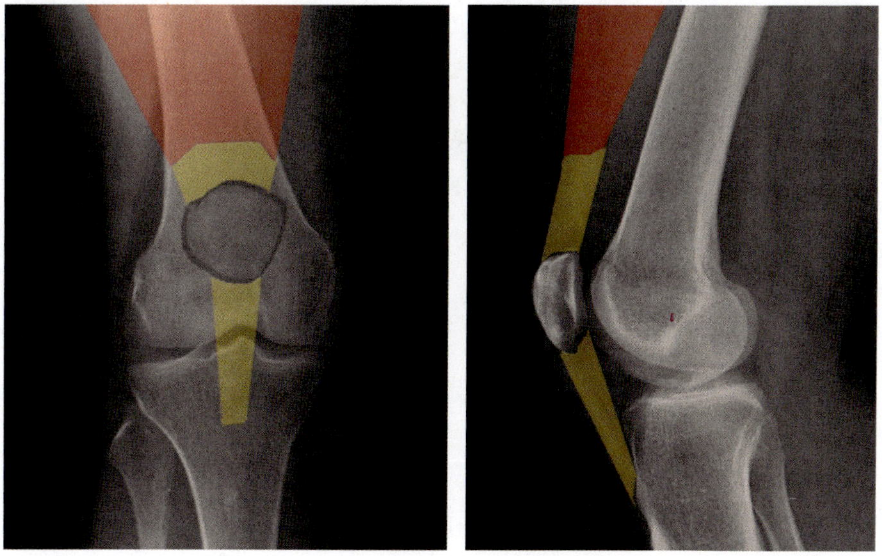

The function of the patella is to increase the distance between the extensor mechanism and the center of rotation of the knee as seen in the sagittal plane. This distance creates a so-called moment arm; the greater the distance, the greater the moment arm and, in turn, the greater the leverage (see Figure 2). Without a patella, the effective strength of knee extension is at least 30% decreased.

Figure 2: As shown by this drawing, extension of the knee is essentially a rotation around the center of the knee in the sagittal plane, powered by the pull of the quads. The greater the distance between the quads and the center of the knee, the longer the lever arm [shown in blue] and thus the greater the torque (rotation force). Without a patella, the pull of the quad is closer to the center of the knee and thus the lever arm is shorter and the force of extension weaker.

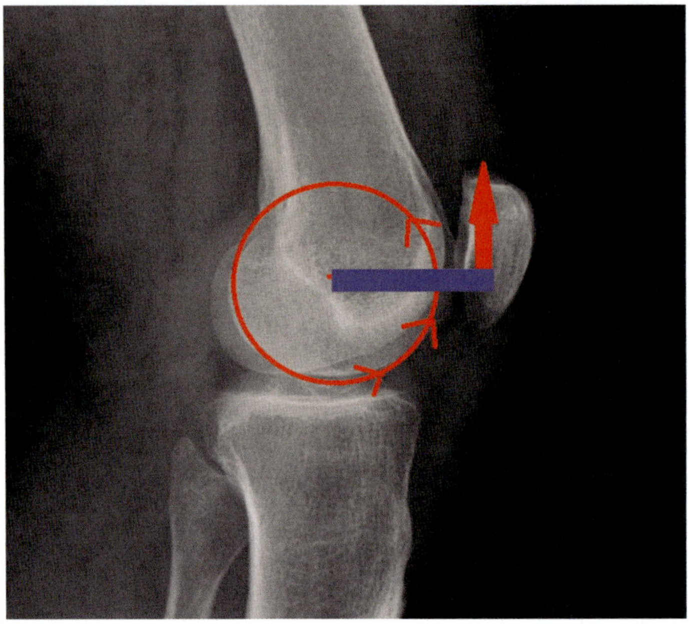

PATIENT PRESENTATION

Tendinopathy

The chief complaint of quadriceps or patellar tendinopathy is pain, localizing to the damaged structure. Because these tendons are directly under the skin there is often little ambiguity if the pain is focal: patients can point and say, "it hurts right there". Tendinopathy can coexist with patellofemoral disorders or bursitis, which sometimes leads to a more nonspecific presentation.

A thorough patient history and physical examination are critical components in diagnosing disorders of the extensor mechanism. Documenting patients' athletic participation as well as whether pain increases with activity are important.

Patients with tendonitis commonly report an insidious onset of sharp anterior knee pain. Patients typically report an increase in pain with activity. Patients may also complain of pain when seated for long periods of time.

Both patellar tendonitis and infrapatellar bursitis are painful to the touch. Patellar tendonitis can be differentiated from infrapatellar bursitis in that the latter condition is painful with side to side pinching of the skin as well (Figure 3A and 3B).

Figure 3A: Direct palpation of the inferior pole of the patella. This is painful if either patellar tendonitis or infrapatellar bursitis is present.

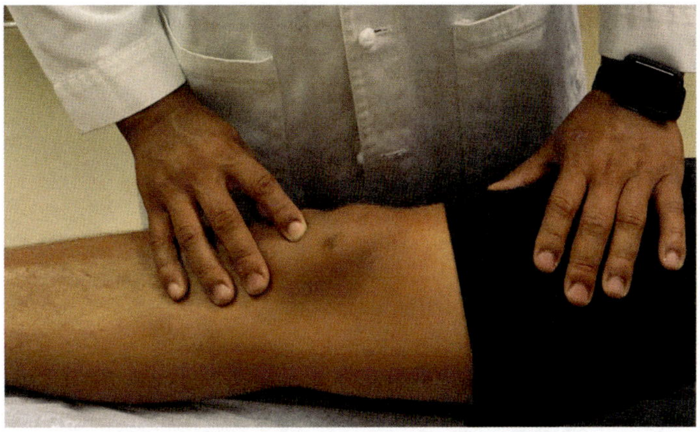

Figure 3B: Pinching the bursa, as shown, will be painful if bursitis is present and not painful if the underlying pathology is deep to that, e.g., in the tendon. If palpation is painful but pinching is not, the diagnosis of tendonitis is likely.

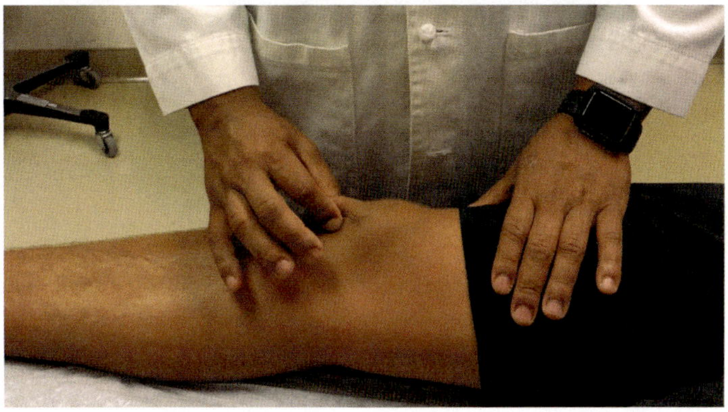

Tendon Rupture

Patients with patellar tendon rupture may report direct trauma (fall) or injury while jumping with the knee bent and the foot planted. Patients will report feeling a tearing or popping sensation at the time of the event.

Quadriceps tendon rupture due to degenerative changes classically presents with a report of a popping or tearing sensation after falling backwards with the foot caught on the ground. Patients may report a history of anterior knee pain before tendon rupture, likely due to tendinopathy. Rupture in athletes typically occurs during eccentric quadriceps contractions, which occur when landing from a jump or changing running directions at high speeds.

Physical exam performed acutely after quadriceps or patellar tendon rupture will reveal swelling and tenderness proximal or distal to the patella, respectively. A palpable defect can often be palpated within the torn tendon.

When either tendon is completely torn patients are unable to extend the knee, perform a straight leg raise, and often cannot bear weight on the injured leg. (That is because in stance phase, the center of gravity of the body is behind the center of rotation of the knee joint and tends therefore to flex it. In ordinary circumstances, the knee does not buckle, and the patient is able to stand upright only because of the resistance to flexion provided by the extensor mechanism.)

When the tendons are partially torn (or if there is sufficient retinacular tissue still intact), patients might still be able to hold the knee in full extension.

OBJECTIVE EVIDENCE

Plain radiographs should be obtained to rule out fractures if the mechanism suggests that one may be present. Radiography can also help identify a soft tissue injury, as a lateral view x-ray will confirm displacement of the patella. A distally displaced patella (patella baja) and a proximally displaced patella (patella alta (see Figure 4) are signs of quadriceps and patellar tendon rupture, respectively.

Figure 4: "Patella alta", that is, a proximally displaced patella, indicates disruption of the infrapatellar ligament. The normal position of the patella is outlined in red. (from https://en.wikipedia.org/wiki/Patellar_tendon_rupture#/media/File:Patellar_tendon_rupture.JPG)

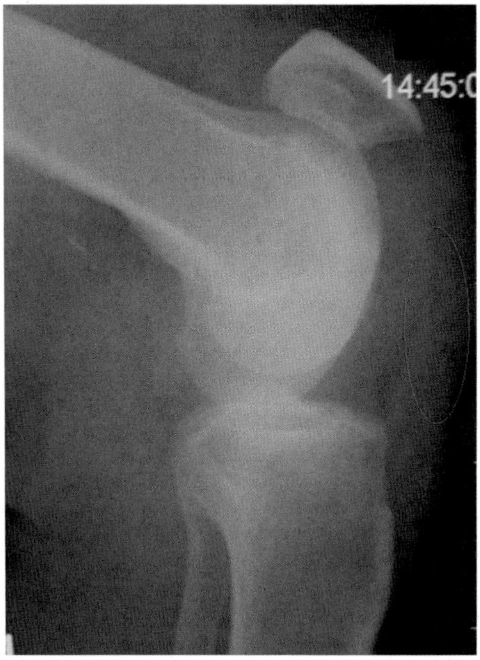

If there is any question whether a disruption is present, an MRI may be helpful. MRI cannot only differentiate between a partial and complete tear, it can localize the injury and provide information about the quality of the surrounding tissue (Figure 5). This latter information may be useful for surgical planning.

Figure 5: MRI showing a quadriceps disruption. (Case courtesy of Dr Ahmed Abdrabou, Radiopaedia.org, rID: 22644)

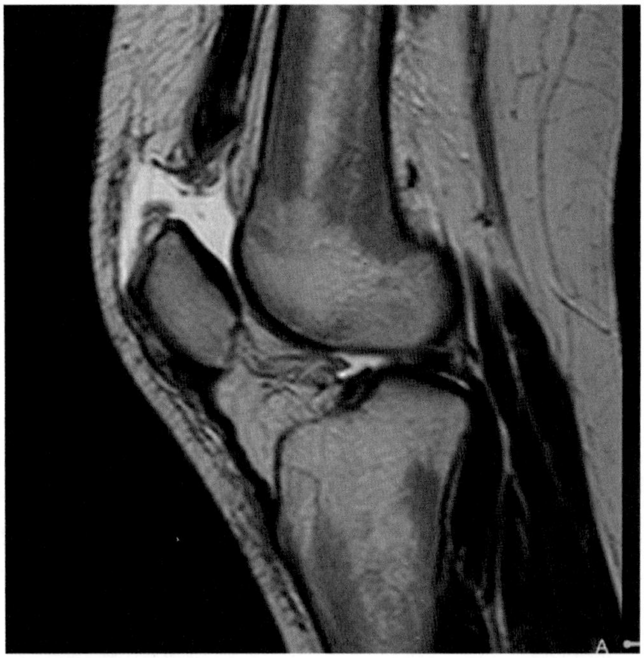

EPIDEMIOLOGY

While quadriceps and patellar tendonitis are common, both quadriceps tendon and patellar tendon ruptures are rare.

Quadriceps tendon rupture occurs predominately in males. Over 80% of tendon ruptures occur in adults over the age of 40 due to degenerative changes; however, younger athletes are also susceptible to tendon rupture due to direct trauma or excessive eccentric joint loading.

Injuries to the patellar tendon are more common in patients under 40 years old. This condition occurs more in jumping athletes, particularly basketball and volleyball players; however, soccer players commonly experience this injury due to the repetitive forces placed on the extensor mechanism. While bilateral rupture for both is possible, patients typically present with unilateral injury, commonly in the dominant leg. Quadriceps ruptures can be seen more commonly in patients with chronic renal disease, patients with diabetes mellitus, or in patients taking steroids for the management of other medical conditions.

DIFFERENTIAL DIAGNOSIS

The differential diagnosis for focal anterior knee pain includes not only tendinopathy but patellofemoral pain syndrome (with or without patellofemoral arthrosis) and bursitis. Of course, these can coexist. A detailed physical examination with imaging can usually differentiate between these diagnoses.

The differential diagnosis for an inability to extend broadly divides into failure of the extensor mechanism or mechanical blockage within the knee joint. These usually can be defined easily by assessing passive motion. A displaced meniscus tear, for example, will impede both active and passive motion, whereas a torn quadriceps will have only limitations on active motion. Incomplete tears, however, may be sufficiently painful that it is difficult to assess passive motion in all instances.

Once it is determined that the extensor mechanism is disrupted, the differential narrows to injuries of the quadriceps tendon, the patella itself and the patellar tendon. Bony injuries in the absence of a direct blow can be assumed absent, though at times patients fall after they tear their tendon making the history a little less clear. X-rays are therefore helpful. Films obtained with the knee in flexion can also indirectly document a soft tissue injury as the patella will be in an abnormal position. Noting the patient's age (again, age over 40 is likely to implicate the quadriceps, and age under 40, the patellar tendon) in addition to performing a physical examination may pinpoint the problem more exactly.

RED FLAGS

In general, tendon injuries do not herald other problems, though the presence of one tendon injury may foreshadow another, and of course tendinopathy itself may suggest an impending rupture.

TREATMENT OPTIONS AND OUTCOMES

Tendinopathy

Because tendinopathy is often an overuse injury, a good first line treatment is relative underuse. Dialing back on activity may allow the body to heal the tendon lesion.

Complete immobilization is not recommended, as this may produce stiffness and atrophy. Physical therapy is intuitively appealing, but there remains no consensus on the best exercises nor the duration of treatment. Nonsteroidal anti-inflammatory drugs (NSAIDs) may also be prescribed; however, these should be reserved for the first 7-14 days after injury as long-term NSAID use has not been proven to be beneficial and may negatively affect tendon healing.

Platelet-rich plasma (PRP) injections have been touted as a promising therapy but as of 2019 have to be labeled as unproven. Steroid injections are not recommended, as they may increase the risk for tendon rupture.

Ice friction massage and isometric flexion stretching may be helpful for patellar tendonitis. (If the knee joint is passively flexed while the patient isometrically contracts the quadriceps, any stretching will be within the patellar tendon itself.)

At times, patellar tendinopathy does not resolve clinically and surgical debridement is indicated.

Non-operative treatment is successful in most patients with tendonitis; however, a small fraction of patients do not respond to non-operative treatment and require surgical debridement. This procedure is successful in more than 75% of cases.

Rupture

For patients with complete rupture of either the quad tendon or patellar tendon, operative repair is indicated to restore normal knee function. That is because even if the tissue were to heal otherwise, the soft tissue will be elongated, and an extensor lag (an inability to fully extend) may result. Also, at the time of operation poor quality tissue can be excised.

In general, surgical repair (Figure 6) uses a midline incision over the knee, and the torn tendon is identified, debrided and secured to bone. (This may use suture anchors or sutures passed through holes drilled within the patella.) Post-operatively, the patient can weight bear with the leg immobilized in extension. Early range of motion exercises are performed, and after 6 weeks the brace is removed and physical therapy is begun. Therapy to strengthen the knee and improve range of motion is continued usually for 3-4 months post-operatively. Full recovery is typically 4-6 months after surgical treatment.

Figure 6: An operative photo showing an open quadriceps repair surgery. The sutures have been passed through tunnel in the patella. (reproduced from PLOS ONE: http://dx.plos.org/10.1371/journal.pone.0194376)

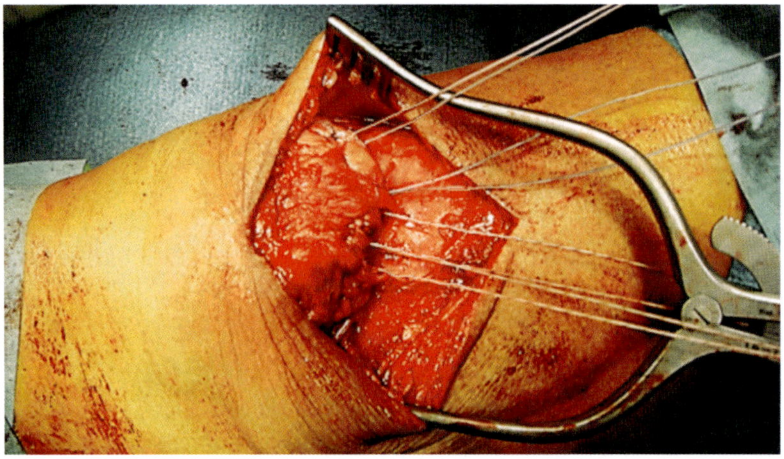

Non-operative management might be reasonable for partial tears of either tendon. Initially patients may be immobilized with the leg in extension for three to six weeks, with weekly follow-up. Immobilization is gradually discontinued when the patient is able to comfortably perform a supine straight leg raise. Physical therapist-guided rehabilitation is instituted to further recovery. Patients should be counseled on the risk of re-injury.

The outcomes following surgical repair for quadriceps and patellar tendon ruptures are good, though often imperfect. Some patients report persistent pain, decreased range of motion and weakness. Nevertheless, by any fair measure, these patients are still markedly better than they would have been without the treatment. (Indeed, the net benefit from surgical treatment of a complete extensor mechanism disruption is among the highest of any orthopedic procedure.)

Delayed operative treatment often leads to worse outcomes.

RISK FACTORS AND PREVENTION

Risk factors for patellar tendon injury include a high body mass index (BMI), a large abdominal circumference, limb-length discrepancy, and flatfoot arch. Weak quadriceps muscles and low flexibility of the quadriceps and hamstring muscles are other factors that may contribute to patellar tendon injury. Additionally, sports involving a lot of jumping, particularly basketball and volleyball, have an increased incidence of patellar tendon injury compared to non-jumping sports.

There are numerous risk factors for degenerative quadriceps tendon rupture including increased age, increased BMI, diabetes mellitus, metabolic syndromes, hyperparathyroidism, polyneuropathy, anabolic steroid abuse, chronic or acute corticosteroid use, and fluoroquinolone use.

MISCELLANY

The patella is a sesamoid bone within the distal tendinous expansion of the extensor mechanism, however it is convenient to think of the quadriceps inserting onto the patella and then the patella itself connecting to the tibia. On this basis, some may consider the patellar tendon to actually be a ligament – soft tissue connecting bone to bone – giving rise to the alternative name for this structure: the infrapatellar ligament.

KEY TERMS

Extensor mechanism, quadriceps muscle, rectus femoris, vastus medialis, vastus lateralis, vastus intermedius, quadriceps tendon, patella and patellar tendon

SKILLS

Recognize the cause of extensor mechanism disruption on plain radiographs. Differentiate between active and passive loss of extension on physical examination, and localize disorders of the extensor mechanism.

CHAPTER 18.

BURSITIS OF THE KNEE

DESCRIPTION

A bursa is a sac-like structure found near joints that allows soft tissues to glide across bony prominences. Bursitis is an inflammation of the bursa. Near the knee, there are three clinically important bursas: the prepatellar (in front of the patella itself), infrapatellar (just distal to the patella) and anserine (on the proximal – medial tibia). Bursitis may result from local injury, infection or systemic diseases such as rheumatoid arthritis or gout. Bursitis due to infection is known as septic bursitis.

STRUCTURE AND FUNCTION

The word bursa (similar to the English word "purse") means sack, though in the healthy state, the sack is mostly empty: that is, the bursa is a double layer of a synovial membrane with a very small amount of synovial fluid between the layers. This anatomical arrangement promotes low friction gliding, and indeed the function of a bursa is to facilitate the gliding of a tendon or ligament around a bony process.

In the knee, there are three bursas (the plural is also spelled "bursae"): the pre-patellar bursa, the infrapatellar bursa and the anserine bursa (Figure 1). As their name implies, the first two bursas are designated by their position relative to the patella. The anserine bursa got its name by its association with the so-called pes anserinus, meaning "foot of the goose", namely, the three tendons that insert onto the anteromedial tibia. (The three tendons are the sartorius, gracilis and semitendinosus.) The pes bursa is typically about 5 cm below the joint line, and therefore symptoms there may be mistaken for articular pathology.

Figure 1: The areas of the pre-patellar (red), infra-patellar (purple) and pes anserine (yellow) bursas are shown.

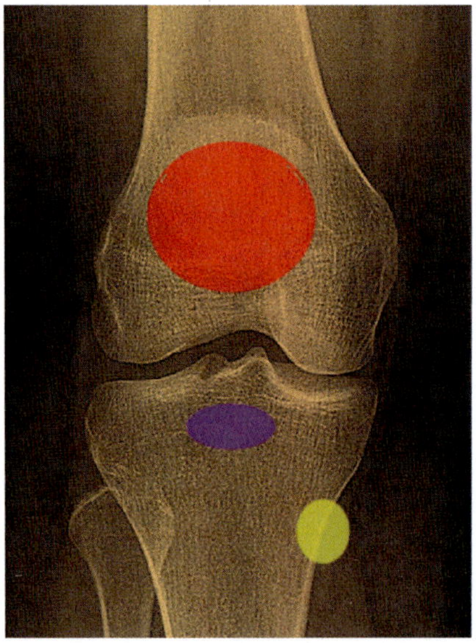

The prepatellar bursa is located superficial to the patella. It decreases friction as the soft tissues glide over the patella during knee flexion and extension. Because of the location of the prepatellar bursa, it is susceptible to repetitive microtrauma, especially when kneeling. Its location also makes it susceptible to blunt and penetrating trauma. Septic prepatellar bursitis can occur following local inoculation due to trauma. The prepatellar bursa has three layers. The subcutaneous layer is located just below the deep dermis and is the one most commonly implicated.

There are two infrapatellar bursae, superficial and deep. The superficial bursa is located between the tibial tubercle and the subcutaneous fascia, while the deep bursa is located between the patellar tendon and the upper tibia.

Infrapatellar bursitis develops in a similar fashion to prepatellar bursitis. Chronic microtrauma secondary to kneeling can lead to superficial bursa wall thickening and inflammation. Chronic overuse and irritation of the patellar tendon can lead to deep infrapatellar bursitis. Its location also makes it susceptible to traumatic causes of bursitis, and septic bursitis.

After injury, synovial cells in the bursa thicken and may undergo villous hyperplasia. Over time, granulation tissue and fibrous tissue may develop. If an inflammatory reaction occurs, the bursa becomes filled with fluid.

PATIENT PRESENTATION

Patients with prepatellar or infrapatellar bursitis typically report a history of chronic kneeling, or a recent increase in time spent kneeling. They may also report difficulty walking and pain that is exacerbated by kneeling. Abrasion of the skin with marked swelling (Figure 2) suggests an infectious etiology.

Figure 2: A clinical photograph of knee bursitis with a skin abrasion and erythema. (from https://upload.wikimedia.org/wikipedia/commons/e/e1/Bursitispraepatellaris.jpg)

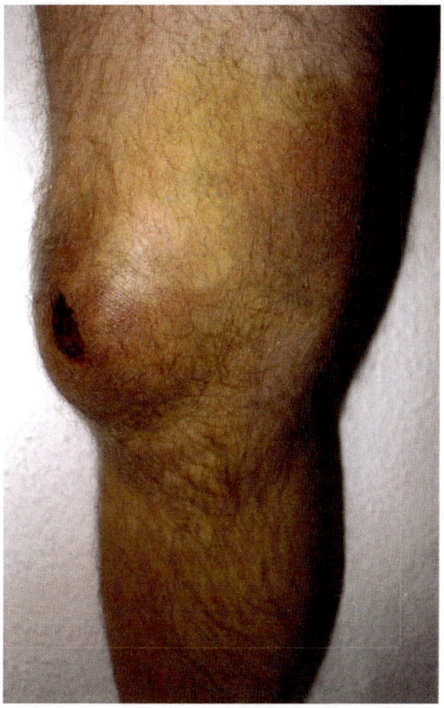

Chronic prepatellar bursitis can present with a soft, non-tender boggy mass on the anterior aspect of the patella, while acute bursitis can present as an erythematous, warm and tender mass. Patients with infrapatellar bursitis exhibit tenderness and edema over the patella tendon. Strength and range of motion are often unaffected but may be limited secondary to pain.

Patients with pes anserine bursitis commonly report medial knee pain that is exacerbated by arising from a seated position or ascending stairs. Patients often do not localize the pes anserine as the source of pain. On exam, patients typically have tenderness near the pes anserine extending to the joint line. The pes anserine is typically 5-7 centimeters below the joint line and 3-4 centimeters medial to the tibial tubercle. Flexion of the knee with the patient supine can help identify the pes anserine. While in this position, if the patient pushes their heels into the table, the gracilis and semitendinosus tendon become more prominent. Resisted knee flexion with the patient lying prone can reproduce symptoms. Hamstring tightness should also be assessed to determine its potential contribution to bursa pain.

OBJECTIVE EVIDENCE

Patients presenting with anterior or medial knee pain should be evaluated with plain radiographs to assess for fractures and presence of osteoarthritis.

Given the soft tissue nature of knee bursitis, radiographs are not helpful in confirming the diagnosis but may reveal a bony prominence that irritates the bursa.

MRI and ultrasound can be useful in localizing soft tissue edema and ruling out other injuries such as MCL or meniscal tears; however, they are not typically required for diagnosis, but if bursitis is present, MRI will detect it (Figure 3).

Figure 3: An MRI of the knee illustrating pre-patellar bursitis (red arrow). (modified from https://radiopaedia.org/articles/prepatellar-bursitis?lang=us)

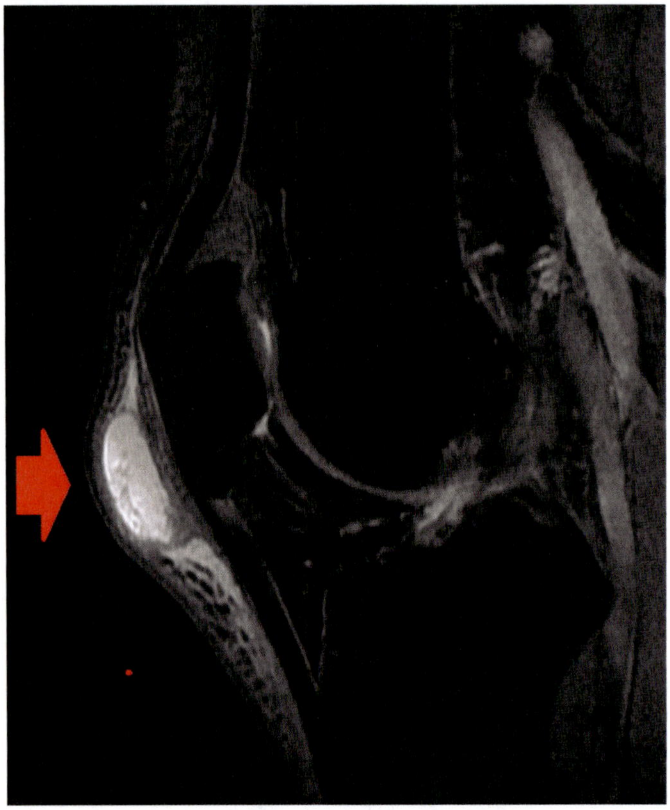

Musculoskeletal ultrasound is emerging as a viable imaging modality to assess the knee joint. Advantages include its ease of availability, economic savings compared to MRI, ability to easily compare abnormalities to the contralateral side, demonstration of fibrillar microanatomy of tendons, ligaments, and muscles, and the ability to compress and dynamically assess structures. Musculoskeletal ultrasound can be utilized to distinguish difficult cases of joint effusion from that of bursal swelling.

Aspiration of an acutely inflamed bursa can help determine if the bursitis is septic in nature.

Non-infectious (aseptic) bursitis is characterized by cell counts lower than 2000/μL. The presence of a predominance of polymorphonuclear leukocytes or a count greater than 5000/μL should be considered indicative of infection.

The fluid should also be examined for monosodium urate crystals (as seen in gout) or calcium pyrophosphate crystals (as seen in pseudogout).

If infection is suspected, the fluid should be sent for Gram stain and culture. Staphylococcus aureus is responsible for about 80% of cases of septic bursitis of the knee.

Varying degrees of inflammation occur in bursitis. The fluid is usually rich in fibrin, but can be hemorrhagic.

A complete blood cell count and blood cultures should be collected if there is concern for systemic infection.

EPIDEMIOLOGY

Bursitis is common: this diagnosis accounts for 0.4% of primary care clinic visits.

The epidemiology of prepatellar bursitis and infrapatellar bursitis are similar. Males have a greater prevalence of prepatellar and infrapatellar bursitis and may be four times more likely to experience bursitis. There is increased prevalence among workers or clergy that spend a significant amount of time kneeling. The prevalence of prepatellar or infrapatellar bursitis is highest amongst construction workers and skilled blue collar workers (painters, plumbers, etc.), approximately 2%. Prepatellar bursitis is also common among wrestlers for the same reason.

Pes anserine bursitis accounts for approximately 2.5% of symptomatic knee evaluations. Pes anserine bursitis affects both young, athletic patients and older patients with knee osteoarthritis. There is also an increased incidence in obese patients, especially females. Interestingly, pes anserine bursitis occurs more frequently in the right knee than in the left knee. Bilateral bursitis occurs in approximately one third of patients.

DIFFERENTIAL DIAGNOSIS

Knee bursitis is one of the many causes of knee pain. Once it is established that there is apparent enlargement of the bursa, the differential diagnosis must separate septic bursitis from noninfectious conditions, and distinguish between bursal inflammation and other soft tissue masses. Septic prepatellar bursitis presents with an acute onset of pain, erythema and focal tenderness. This may follow a history of trauma or cellulitis. Notably, a long-standing bursa can be, acutely infected. A soft tissue mass, such as a lipoma, can present as a firm non-tender, non-erythematous mass on the anterior aspect of the knee. Cellulitis can present with erythema and pain. Often, there is a known history of trauma to the skin. This may be confused with acute septic bursitis. Cellulitis has limited edema and typically spreads, while bursitis remains limited to the bursa.

It is important to recall that many patients with pes bursitis will also have medial compartment arthritis, and therefore it becomes important to distinguish between bursal pain and true joint pain. Bursal pain may be most amenable to physical therapy and medication; detecting the bursa as a source of the pain may prevent overtreatment of the underlying arthritis.

Infrapatellar bursitis may present with symptoms that are indistinguishable from those caused by patellar tendinitis. Fortunately, the treatment of the two is roughly the same and therefore they may not need to be precisely differentiated.

RED FLAGS

Patients with fever, severe knee pain, inability to bear weight and significantly limited range of motion should be evaluated for a septic joint or septic prepatellar bursitis. Patients with systemic symptoms such as fevers, chills, night sweats, and tachycardia should be evaluated for a systemic infection (sepsis).

TREATMENT OPTIONS AND OUTCOMES

Treatment options for knee bursitis include benign neglect ("observation"), weight loss, non-steroidal anti-inflammatory medication (NSAIDs), physical therapy, aspiration with or without corticosteroid injections, immobilization and in rare instances operative treatment.

Extracorporeal shock wave therapy and kinesio-taping have also been investigated as potential treatments but are not commonly utilized.

Generally, non-septic bursitis is a self-limited condition. Treatment is best focused on addressing the inciting condition to prevent recurrence.

In the case of pes anserine bursitis, observation alone is usually not an effective approach. That is because bursitis in this location is commonly due to an underlying condition such as obesity or muscular tightness. Until the underlying cause is addressed, the bursitis will persist. Weight loss can help alleviate the symptoms of pes anserine bursitis. NSAIDs are used when tolerated to decrease bursa inflammation and pain. Physical therapy can decrease pes anserine symptoms by stretching the hamstring muscles, thus relieving pressure on the bursa. Physical therapy also focuses on strengthening the quadriceps and other knee stabilizing muscles.

Corticosteroid injected directly into the bursa can relieve symptoms by decreasing the inflammatory response. Like NSAIDs, corticosteroids can be used in conjunction with other treatment to increase efficacy.

Unlike pes anserine bursitis, prepatellar and infrapatellar bursitis can be treated with lifestyle modification and the use of knee pads. NSAIDs can be used to decrease inflammation; however, corticosteroid injections are generally avoided due to the risk of infection in prepatellar and infrapatellar bursitis. In the case of chronic prepatellar bursitis, corticosteroid injection can be used if other treatment modalities have failed.

Patients with septic bursitis are treated with antibiotics, splint immobilization, and urgent bursal aspiration. Aspiration may be repeated if the fluid re-accumulates. These patients may require surgical debridement if antibiotic treatment and aspiration of the bursa is not successful.

Operative bursectomy may be utilized also for cases of intractable non-infectious bursitis.

There is limited published data about the outcomes of knee bursitis treatments. Most patients treated with oral or topical NSAID experience significant symptom relief. Both physical therapy and corticosteroid injection significantly improve pain and symptoms secondary to pes anserine bursitis. Approximately 70% of patients treated with steroid injections will experience significant improvement, and 30-91% will experience resolution of symptoms.

Extracorporeal shock wave therapy is more effective than placebo for pes anserine bursitis symptom relief. Kinesio-taping for pes anserine bursitis may be superior to naproxen combined with physical therapy for both pain and tissue swelling relief.

Surgical bursectomy is an effective treatment for persistent bursitis; up to 80% of patients will have complete resolution of symptoms and return to pre-injury work and activities. However, patients with jobs that require significant kneeling or with chronic prepatellar bursitis may continue to be symptomatic.

RISK FACTORS AND PREVENTION

Valgus knee deformity, obesity, diabetes, and female sex are risk factors for pes anserine bursitis. The risk for pes anserine bursitis can be decreased by stretching the hamstring muscles as well as strengthening the quadriceps and secondary knee stabilizing muscles. Maintenance of a healthy weight can also decrease the risk of pes anserine bursitis.

Blue collar employment, significant kneeling, and male sex are risk factors for prepatellar and infrapatellar bursitis. The risk of prepatellar and infrapatellar bursitis can be reduced by the use of knee pads when kneeling for an extended period of time and activity modification when possible.

MISCELLANY

Prepatellar bursitis is commonly known as housemaid's knee. Housemaids would injure this bursa due to frequent kneeling when cleaning.

Infrapatellar bursitis is commonly known as clergyman's knee. Clergyman injured this bursa by commonly kneeling on hard surfaces while in prayer.

The university financial officer is called "bursar", for in the old days, he (and it always was a "he") carried the college's sack of coins.

KEY TERMS

Knee bursitis, pes anserine, patella, inflammation

SKILLS

Identify bursas on exam by palpation of key lower extremity anatomical landmarks. Recognize septic bursitis.

CHAPTER 19.

PATELLOFEMORAL DISORDERS

DESCRIPTION

Anterior knee pain may be found with patellar instability (subluxation or complete dislocation of the patella out of the trochlear groove) or patellofemoral arthrosis. It may also have no objectively defined cause, in which case the label "patellofemoral pain syndrome" is applied. Many patients with patellofemoral pain syndrome improve with no treatment. Patellar instability may be treated with muscle strengthening therapy or braces; at times, however, surgery is needed.

STRUCTURE AND FUNCTION

The patellofemoral joint is formed by the patella and the anterior surface of the distal femur, an area called the trochlear groove.

The patella is a sesamoid bone that is embedded within the quadriceps tendon and serves to increase the mechanical advantage of the quadriceps muscle. The undersurface of the patella is composed of two main facets, lateral and medial. The lateral facet is longer and less steep, matching the geometry of the lateral aspect of the trochlea.

Figure 1: A sunrise view of the patella, showing the patella sitting within the trochlear groove of the femur. (from http://www.wikiradiography.net/page/the+skyline+patella+projection)

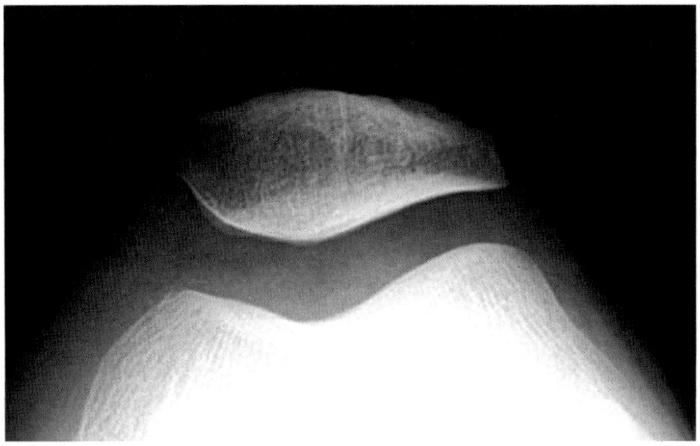

Stability of the patella in the patellofemoral joint relies on normal trochlear morphology of the femur. The trochlear groove must be sufficiently deep to hold the patella, especially in flexion. Stability also depends on the alignment of the tibia relative to the femur. A so-called valgus or "knock-knee" alignment of the knee joint increases the lateral vector of the quadriceps. If the lateral vector is too great, the quadriceps can pull the patella out of the trochlear groove, especially as the knee nears terminal extension. This can be assessed by two measurements: the angle between the quadriceps and the infrapatellar ligament, so-called Q angle and the tibial tubercle to trochlear groove (TT-TG) distance (Figure 2).

Figure 2: Q-angle: The Q angle is defined by a line from the anterior-superior iliac spine through the midpoint of the patella and another line from the tibial tuberosity through the midpoint of the patella. The line from the anterior-superior iliac spine through the midpoint of the patella represents the pull of the quadriceps. This force vector, shown by the green line in the enlarged view, can be resolved into a superior force (red line) and laterally-directed force (blue line). Thus, the greater the Q angle, the greater force pulling the patella laterally, out of its healthy position in the trochlea.

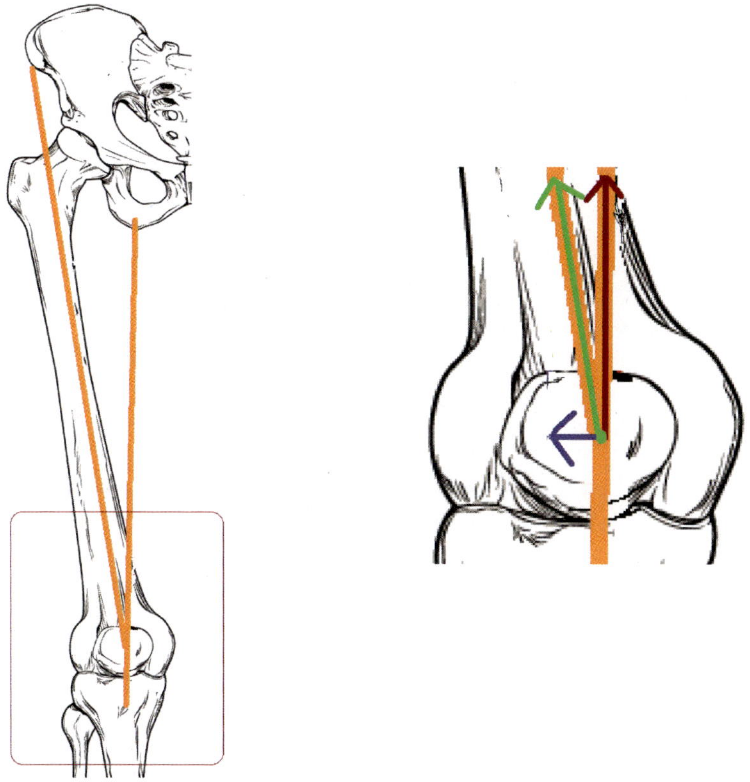

Figure 3: The tibial tubercle to trochlear groove distance is defined by 2 slices of a CT scan. First, the base of the trochlea is defined, and line is drawn through it, down to the bottom on the scan. The position of this (red) line is identified by the star on a line denoting medial-to-lateral distance (shown in blue). On a more distal slice, the tibial tubercle is identified, and a line is drawn through it down to the bottom of the scan as well, shown here in green, and the position is also identified. The distance between these two lines is the tibial tubercle to trochlear groove distance. (Redrawn from a case courtesy of Dr. Ayush Goel, Radiopaedia.org, rID: 28749)

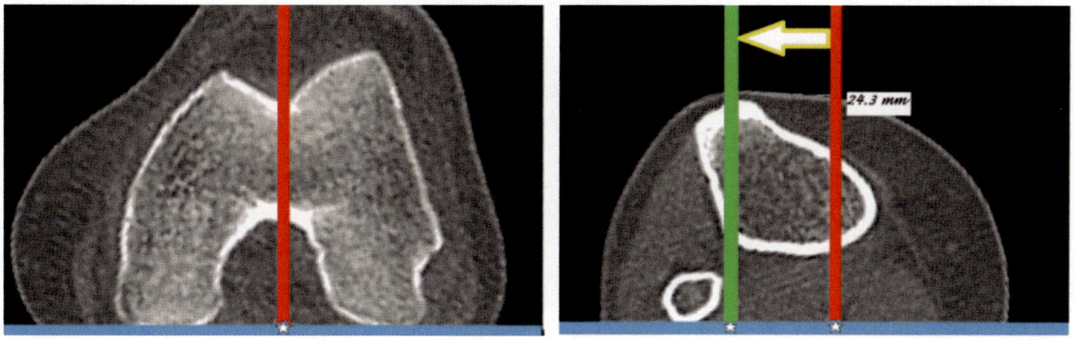

Additional static stability is provided by the lateral retinaculum, medial retinaculum, medial patellofemoral ligament, and medial patella-tibial ligament.

The vastus medialis obliquus provides dynamic stability, actively pulling the patella medially, to keep it located within the joint (Figure 4).

Figure 4: As shown, the pull of the vastus medialis obliquus (red line) has a medially-directed component (white arrow), which tends to stabilize the patella. Weakness or atrophy of this muscle is thus associated with patellofemoral disorders.

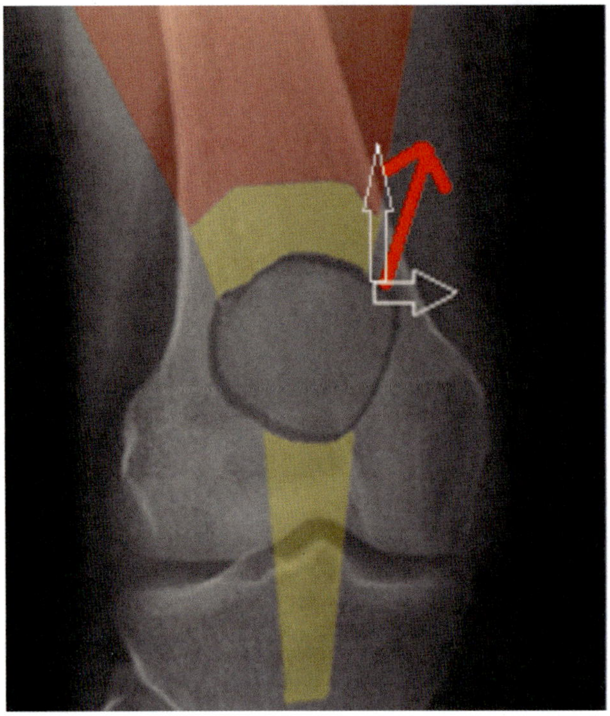

During initial knee flexion (<30 degrees), the major restraints to lateral translation and dislocation are the soft tissue structures; beyond 30 degrees, the bony structures are the primary determinants of stability.

The medial patellofemoral ligament is the primary soft tissue restraint against lateral translation of the patella. This ligament is torn when there is excessive lateral translation of the patella.

In cases of so-called patella alta, a longer than normal patellar tendon allows the patella to rest more proximally. As a result, the patella does not enter the trochlear groove until higher-than-normal levels of knee flexion have occurred. In patients with recurrent instability, trochlear dysplasia has been noted to be present in up to 96% of patients.

PATIENT PRESENTATION

A thorough patient history and physical examination are critical components in diagnosing patellofemoral pain syndrome and patellar instability. Patients will report pain and possibly swelling in their knee with increasing intensity such as climbing or descending stairs, squatting, running, jumping, or "cutting" during sports activities.

In some cases of patellofemoral pain syndrome, patients will commonly report feeling pain "behind," "underneath," or "around" the patella. Many patients will not experience swelling with patellofemoral pain syndrome; however, patients will note stiffness, particularly when the knee is flexed, as well as potentially "popping" or "catching" sensations.

Patients may also note overall weakness in their leg as well as a feeling that their knee might "give way" again in cases of patellar instability. Discoloration medially and pain along the medial aspect of the knee are commonly seen. The number of prior identifiable dislocations and subluxation episodes for the patient as well as any history of ligamentous laxity or dislocation of family members must be noted.

Physical examination should note alignment and range of motion; the presence or absence of tenderness should be noted as well.

Examination maneuvers are shown in the figures 5-8.

Figure 5: The Patellar glide and tilt test: With the patient lying in the supine position and the knee extended, the patella is grasped and first translated medially (green arrow), and displacement is measured in quadrants. Displacement of less than one quadrant medially indicates tightness of the lateral structures, whereas hypermobility is indicated by displacement of more than three quadrants. The examiner next uses the thumb, touching the lateral side of the patella, in an attempt to tilt the patella from its resting position (red arrow). The patella should "tilt" back to at least the neutral (equatorial) position, i.e., the medial and lateral facets are parallel to the exam table.

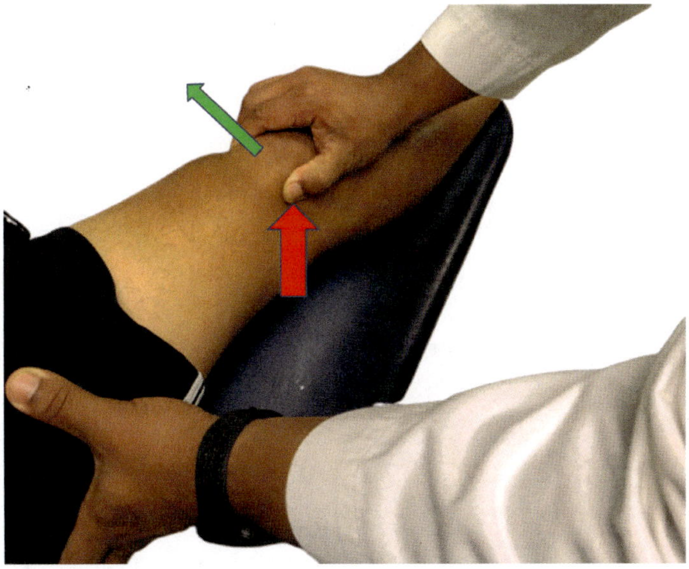

(Note that these maneuvers are performed in sequence, not simultaneously. For the two tests, the position of the patient and the examiner are the same, with the only difference being the motion of the examiner's thumb, hence a single photo is shown. These test do address a unified issue: namely, can the patella be moved passively a "normal" amount?)

Figure 6: Patellar inhibition: in the presence of arthrosis, a patient will not want to load the damaged area, and will actually shut off ("inhibit") the quadriceps if that muscle is forcing the contact. This can be elicited by asking the patient to kick out (purple curved arrow) against resistance (red arrow). Subtle relative weakness suggests inhibition and in turn arthrosis of the patellofemoral joint. (Because a different point of the patella articulates in different degrees of flexion, the best way to assess patellar inhibition is to have the patient actively extend the knee against resistance at 30, 45, 60 and 90 degrees of flexion.)

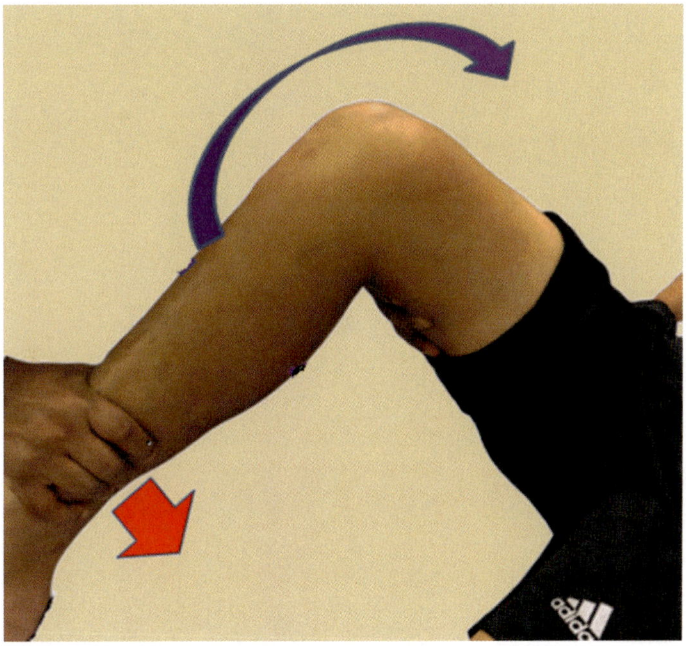

Figure 7: Patellar apprehension: the examiner tries to push the patella out of the trochlea with the knee extended. A reported sense of impending dislocation ("apprehension") is a positive test.

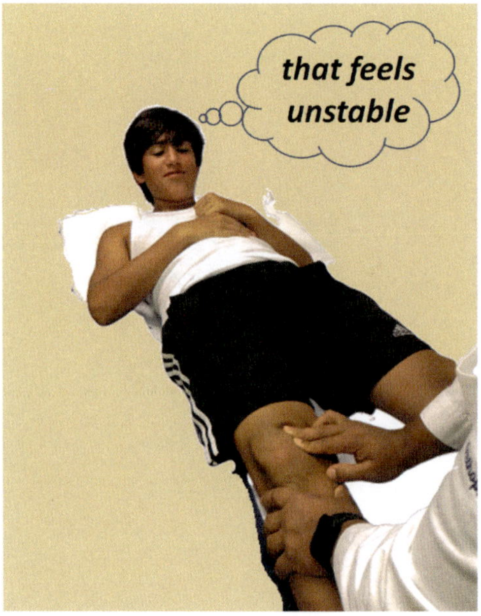

Figure 8: Patellar tracking (J-sign): The examiners scrutinizes the position of the patella when the knee moves from full flexion (top panel) to mid-flexion (middle panel) and then extension (bottom panel). In full flexion, the patella, outlined in red, will be located in the trochlea groove even if the soft tissues are lax; but in the setting of laxity, the patella will move to a lateral position in extension. Thus, if the soft tissues are lax, the patella will follow a "J" or "L" course when the knee moves from flexion to extension, or vice versa (left vs right). In the figure, the model is normal, and no "J" sign is demonstrated: the patella remains central.

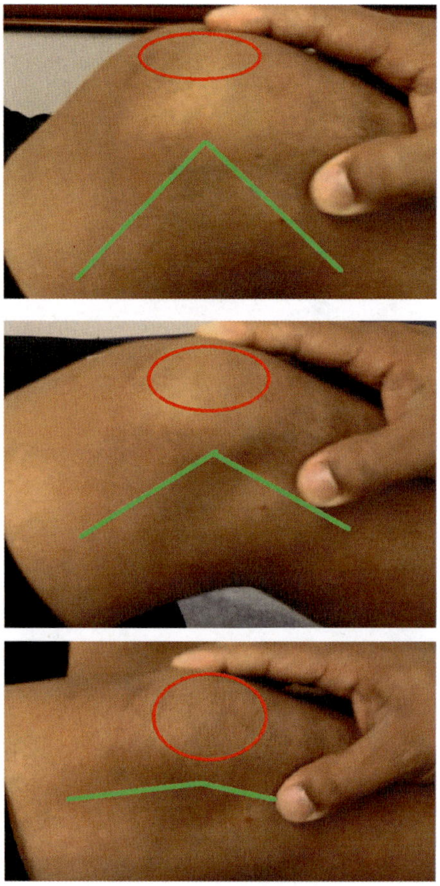

Most patella dislocations occur laterally; therefore, the lateral patellar apprehension test represents the best test for determining patellar instability.
The quadriceps and patellar tendons should be palpated to detect tendinosis.

Additionally, a Lachman's test, pivot shift, anterior and posterior drawer test, dial test, and varus/valgus stress test should be performed to rule out other injuries.

OBJECTIVE EVIDENCE

Patellofemoral pain syndrome is primarily a clinical diagnosis and can be made without radiographic imaging. Nevertheless, x-rays will commonly be ordered to rule out structural abnormalities.

In cases of suspected patella instability, anteroposterior and posteroanterior 45° weight bearing views should be obtained to examine any abnormal anatomy, particularly current presence of dislocation. Lateral radiographs should be ordered to examine patella height, trochlear dysplasia and patellar tilt.

The sunrise view (Figure 9) can evaluate for lateral subluxation and patellar tilt.

Figure 9: In this sunrise view, the normal patellofemoral joint is shown on the x-ray, with the red line outlining patellar tilt (rotation of medial side up) as well as lateral subluxation. Both contribute to excess compression laterally.

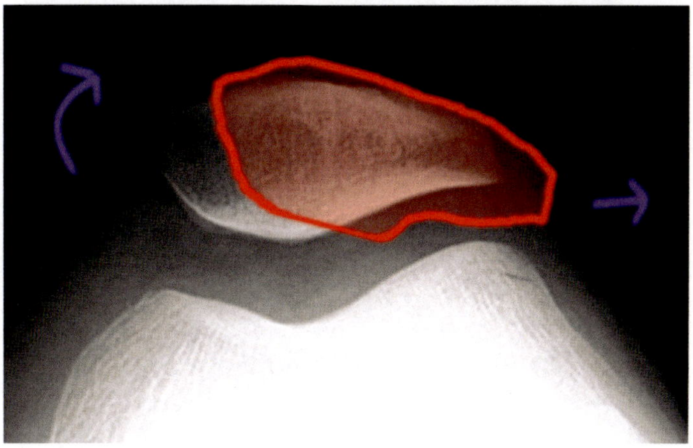

CT scans provide valuable axial information allowing evaluation of the anterior tubercle to trochlear groove distance. The mean tibial tubercle to trochlear groove distance has been noted to be 9 mm while a tibial tubercle to trochlear groove distance of 20 mm or more has a 90% association with patellar instability. CT is more reliable than MRI for this assessment.

MRI is valuable in assessing for cartilage/osteochondral injury as well as soft tissue structures of the knee. MRI will help evaluate any articular cartilage damage on the medial facet of the patella and bone bruising of the lateral femoral condyle.

Figure 10: MRI of an acute patellar dislocation. Edema is seen in both the patella and the lateral condyle, reflecting the impact ("kissing contusion") between these bones when the patella dislocated laterally. The red lightning bolt points to the disrupted medial patellofemoral ligament, whereas the lateral ligament is intact (blue star). (Case courtesy of Dr. Hector RiveraMelo, Radiopaedia.org, rID: 27014)

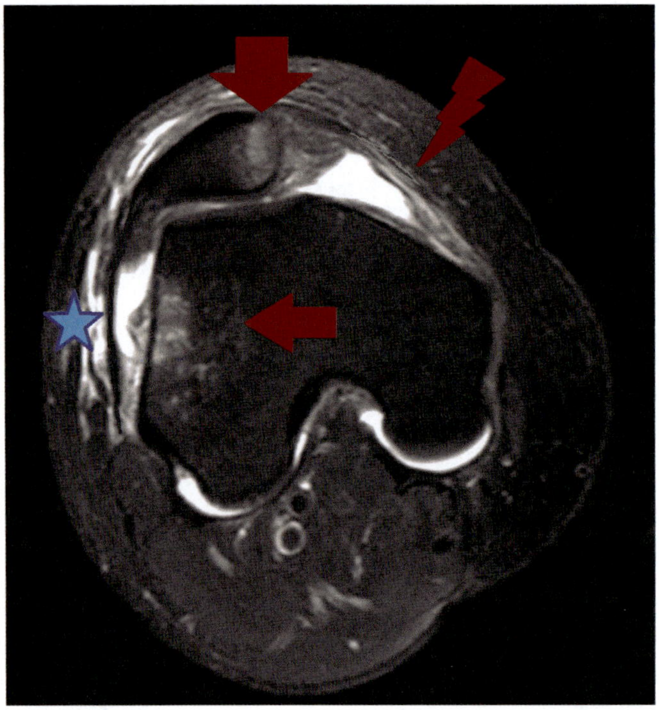

EPIDEMIOLOGY

Anterior knee pain is the most common knee diagnosis in sports medicine centers and among runners. Up to 11% of musculoskeletal complaints in the outpatient setting are caused by anterior knee pain, most commonly patellofemoral pain syndrome, and the incidence of patellofemoral pain syndrome in runners is between 16% and 25%.

The majority of patellar instability occurs in young, active individuals with an incidence of 1 per 1000 people. Overall, patellar dislocations represent approximately 3% of all knee injuries. Females are more likely to have patellar dislocations than men and the most commonly affected age group is individual's ages 10 to 16 years old. Patellar instability is commonly traumatic in nature due to either contact or non-contact mechanisms; however, patients with patellar malalignment may experience frequent low-energy patellar dislocations.

DIFFERENTIAL DIAGNOSIS

Anterior knee pain may be due to instability (with or without an overt history of dislocation); it may be due to patellofemoral arthrosis (with or without radiographic confirmation); it may be due to tendinosis on either side of the patella; or it may have no known causes.

At times, patellar dislocations reduce spontaneously, such that the patient may not be aware that the patella dislocated other than feeling a shift in their knee.

Patients may report buckling due to patellar inhibition, but of course true ligamentous laxity must be excluded before that diagnosis is credited.

RED FLAGS

Gross laxity of the patellofemoral stabilizers may suggest a connective tissue disorder, such as Ehlers-Danlos syndrome.

Incomplete passive motion after a patellofemoral dislocation suggests a loose body within the knee.

TREATMENT OPTIONS AND OUTCOMES

For patients diagnosed with patellofemoral pain syndrome, a comprehensive rehabilitation program is the first line of treatment. Rehabilitation programs should include modification or cessation of activities as well as physical therapy.

A knee sleeve, splint, or taping may be used as well. This may help hold the patella within the trochlea. Alternatively, these may help simply by serving to remind the patient to avoid full flexion.

Recovery from patellofemoral pain syndrome can take longer than most patients anticipate.

Patients with pain but without a correctable anatomic lesion are rarely helped (and may be hurt) by surgery.

Patients sustaining their first dislocation can be treated with a brace. However, even in first time dislocations (especially if there is a large hematoma that raises concern for osteochondral injury) – an MRI is useful. This test can detect loose bodies and assess for any damage to the ligaments and cartilage.

After a first-time dislocation, physical therapy (PT) is started 1-2 weeks after the dislocation, to help achieve normal range of motion and strength and is continued for 2-3 months. In some cases, 4-5 months of PT is necessary in order for athletes to return to their pre-injury level of activity.

In cases of recurrent instability, operative treatment is frequently recommended. Operative treatment is based upon the patient's anatomy and the spectrum of injury. It may consist of either an isolated soft tissue procedure or a bony realignment procedure or both.

The most common procedure is reconstruction of the medial patellofemoral ligament with an autograft (hamstring tendon) or allograft. Although less common, repair of the medial patellofemoral ligament is possible in some patients who seek treatment promptly and have a bony avulsion of the ligament from the medial aspect of the patella.

In cases of recurrent instability where the distance between the tibial tubercle and the trochlear groove is greater than 20 mm, an osteotomy of the tibial tubercle is needed. In this operation, the tubercle is moved medially, to realign the patellar tendon and in turn make the patella track more medially.

For patients with an open growth plate, surgeons will commonly perform an isolated soft tissue procedure and then perform the realignment surgery after closure of the growth plates to prevent further cartilage damage underneath the kneecap as well as to prevent arthritis from developing.

In cases of extreme dysplasia, operations to deepen the base of the trochlea or elevate the lateral facet (so-called trochleoplasty procedures) may be performed. This approach has not gained widespread acceptance among orthopaedic surgeons.

For either procedure, rehabilitation typically lasts 4-6 months post-surgery and final recovery and return to sports is not usually achieved until after 6 months from reconstruction (when full range of motion, stability, and strength have been restored).

Following completion of a thorough rehabilitation program, patellofemoral pain syndrome commonly resolves–but to prevent recurrence, appropriate conditioning of the muscles around the knee, particularly the quadriceps and the hamstrings is essential.

After an initial dislocation, the ligaments are stretched from the injury; therefore, patients are at an increased risk for either a recurrent subluxation or dislocation. The incidence of recurrent instability following conservative treatment has been noted to be between 15% and 44%. After a second dislocation, the risk of recurrence increases to over 50% and in younger patients (less than 25 years of age, particularly those with open growth plates) the risk of recurrence after a second dislocation has been noted to be as high as 70%.

Following operative treatment, the success rate for stabilization has been noted to be as high as 85% – 90% for both soft tissue and bony procedures.

RISK FACTORS AND PREVENTION

Risk factors for patellofemoral pain syndrome include females and young adults as the condition is commonly referred to as "runner's knee", due to the high occurrence in athletes. Additionally, malalignment of the kneecap and overuse from vigorous athletics or training are also significant risk factors.

For patellar instability, risk factors include young age (under the age of 25 with a peak incidence between ages 10-16 years old) and open growth plates (this is particularly a risk factor for patients after primary dislocation). A prior history or patellar dislocation or subluxation represents a significant risk factor as up to 44% of patients treated conservatively may experience a second instability episode.

KEY TERMS

Patellar dislocation, patellar subluxation, medial patellofemoral ligament injury, Q-angle, tibial tubercle to trochlear groove distance, trochlear dysplasia, patella alta

SKILLS

Perform Patellar, tilt, apprehension and inhibition tests. Assess Q angle on imaging.

CHAPTER 20.

MENISCUS TEARS

DESCRIPTION

The medial and lateral meniscus (plural: menisci) are crescent-shaped pieces of fibrocartilage that lie atop the tibia to cushion its contact with the femur and help stabilize the knee. Because these functions subject the menisci to high forces, the menisci are subject to tearing. Both acute traumatic events and simple degeneration can be responsible for tearing. Many patients with degenerative tears of the meniscus have no symptoms, though some have focal joint line pain or a sense of catching. The menisci themselves have very little intrinsic capacity for healing, and thus persistently symptomatic tears are treated with partial meniscectomy (removal), though tears near the capsule can be repaired.

STRUCTURE AND FUNCTION

The medial and lateral menisci are thin pieces of fibrocartilage that sit atop the tibial plateau (Figure 1). The menisci are C-shaped when viewed in profile, tapering from about 5mm in height near the capsule to a central edge.

Figure 1: An axial view of the medial (red) and lateral (blue) meniscus atop the tibial plateau. The articular cartilage that is not covered by the menisci is shown in yellow, and the (cut) cruciate ligaments are shown in purple. (Modified from Gray's Anatomy, https://en.wikipedia.org/wiki/Meniscus_(anatomy)#/media/File:Gray349.png)

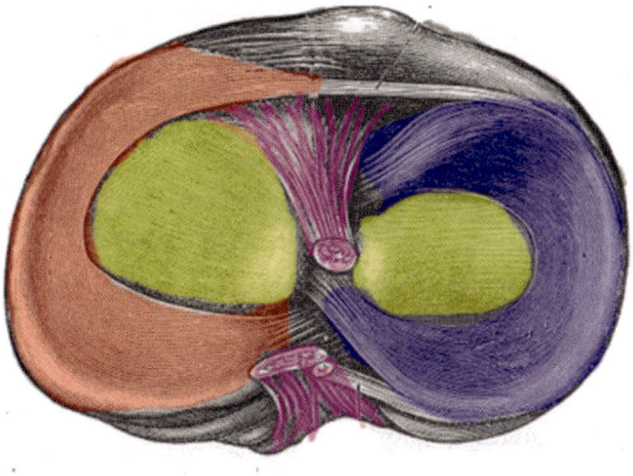

The menisci also help lubricate the knee joint. Beyond that, the meniscus is thought to have three mechanical functions. First, it allows the rounded femoral condyle to make broader contact with the tibia, thereby dissipating pressure. (Because pressure is equal to force/area, greater area leads to lower pressure for a given force) (Figure 2).

Figure 2: As shown on the left, in this lateral view schematic, the rounded femoral condyle has only a small area of contact with the flatter tibial plateau. With the triangular menisci in place, the area of contact is greatly increased, leading to lower contact pressures, as the force is dissipated over a broader surface.

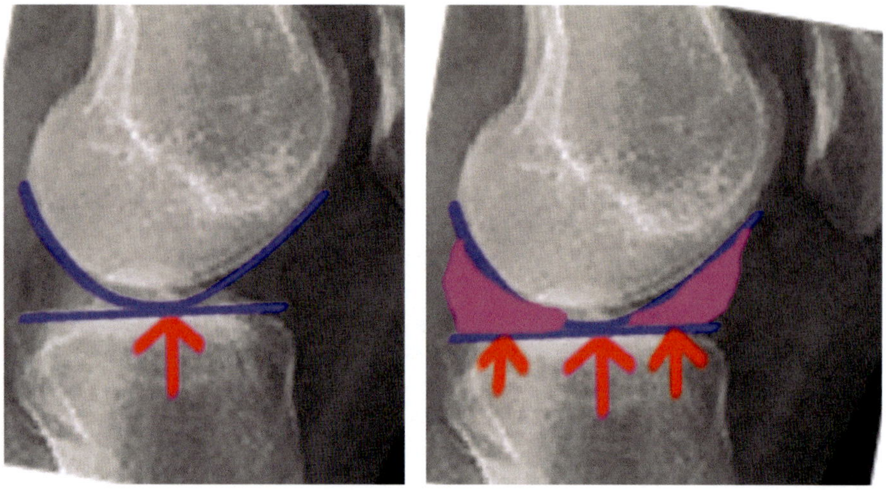

In addition, because the menisci are more elastic than articular cartilage, they also function as shock absorbers.

Last, the menisci (especially on the medial side) help stabilize the knee, by a so-called chock block effect (Figure 3).

Figure 3: As shown in the x-ray to the left, the femoral condyle (black curved line) abuts the posterior horn of the meniscus (orange). As such, the meniscus can stabilize the knee in the same way a wheel chock next to a tire can prevent a vehicle from rolling, as shown in the figure to the right.

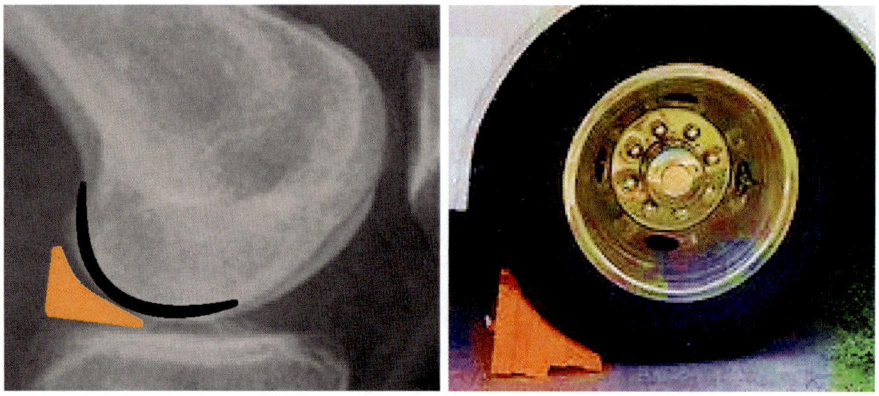

There are some important differences between the medial and lateral meniscus. The medial meniscus is more firmly attached to the tibial condyle by the deep medial collateral ligament (MCL); the lateral meniscus is relatively mobile. Thus, the medial meniscus is a more important stabilizer. Because the medial meniscus is tethered, it is also more susceptible to injury and is torn approximately three times more often than the lateral meniscus.

The lateral meniscus is separated from the capsule at the popliteal hiatus, an aperture through which the popliteus tendon courses into the joint.

Only the most peripheral part (about 3 mm) of the menisci have blood vessels and thus meniscal tears have little inherent capacity to heal. Because the blood supply enters from the capsule at the periphery (the so-called red zone), some tears there might heal; central tears (called "white zone" tears owing to the lack of blood supply) are thought to have no healing potential.

The menisci also have no pain sensors within them. Thus, to the extent that meniscal tears are painful (and many are) it is due to irritation of the nearby synovium or capsule.

PATIENT PRESENTATION

Traumatic tears of a healthy meniscus normally occur in active young adults who present with pain and swelling after an acute event. A classic report is a twisting injury with the foot planted and the knee flexed, though this is certainly not required.

There may be an effusion of variable size. Pain typically localizes to the joint line. Incomplete range of passive motion suggests a displaced tear. A displaced tear usually blocks the final 20 degrees of terminal extension, with reasonably free motion in the flexion arc beyond that. Although some motion is possible, this condition is termed "locking" – though "blocking" may be a more apt word.

Meniscal tears can be seen in conjunction with other injuries (such as a tear of the anterior cruciate ligament) and the presentation may be dominated by that other condition.

Degenerative tears normally are found in adults over the age of 40. The presentation is similar to that of arthritis, but the pain from the meniscus is more likely to be focally on the joint line, with or without mechanical symptoms such as catching.

The physical exam must note the pattern of gait, alignment, range of motion and the presence of an effusion. Integrity of the ligaments must also be assessed.

There are specific tests for diagnosing a meniscal tear on examination, but all are based on subjective responses. The best test is assessing for joint line tenderness (Figure 4). This too is subjective, but it is simple. Tenderness above or below the joint line suggests that a meniscal tear is not responsible for symptoms.

Figure 4: Tenderness precisely on the joint line is more specific for meniscal pathology. The tenderness associated with arthritis often extends to the bone above or below. The joint line can be found by tracing the contours of the bones with gentle finger pressure while flexing/extending the knee passively and sensing the movement of the tibia relative to the femur. (The medial joint line is shown here.)

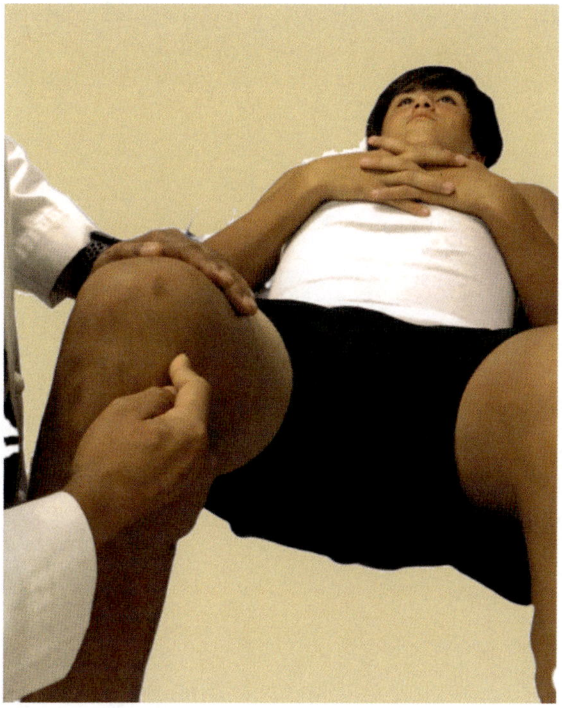

OBJECTIVE EVIDENCE

MRI is the gold standard in terms of accurately diagnosing a meniscus tear. A meniscal tear will manifest as increased signal within the meniscus that extends to the tibial or femoral articular surface (Figures 5 and 6). Signal change confined within the meniscus itself (that is, the signal change that does not cross the triangular borders of the meniscal surfaces) represents internal degenerative change.

Figure 5: The MRI appearance of a medial meniscal tear is shown here. (Case courtesy of A. Prof Frank Gaillard, Radiopaedia.org, rID: 6361)

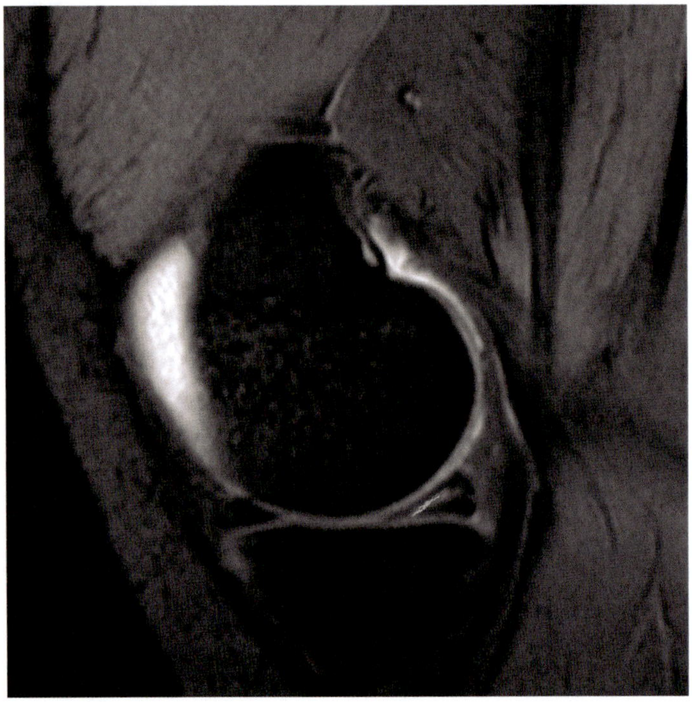

Figure 6: An arthroscopy photo of a medial meniscal tear. A metal probe (seen coursing from roughly the 7 O'clock position towards 1 O'clock) is placed in the tear and pulled forward (red arrow). As shown here, the probe is able to displace the free edge of the torn meniscus into the joint space. This displacement, which can occur during normal knee motion, is thought to be the source of symptoms. The displaced fragment can cause a catching sensation, but also by tugging on the remaining meniscus, can irritate the (very sensitive) capsule to which the meniscus is attached at the periphery.

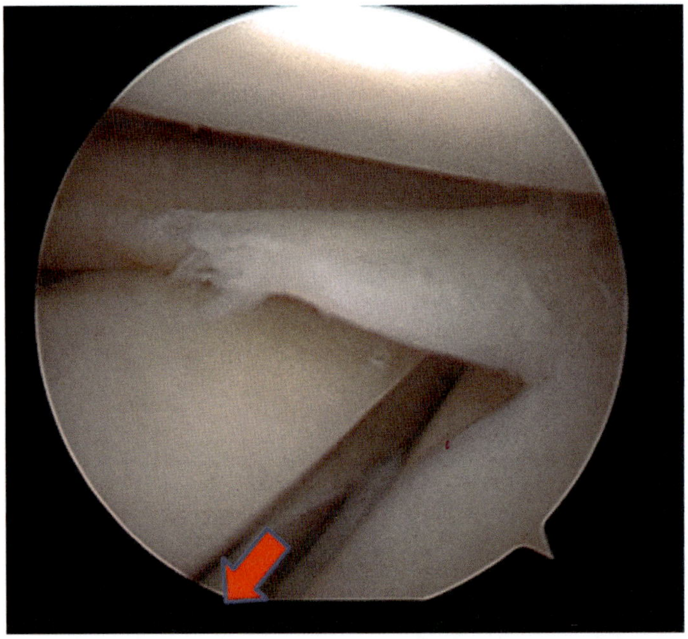

The use of MRI is perhaps best understood by reminding oneself that it is a diagnostic test, and like all such tests, should be used if and only if the results could affect the treatment of the patient. Contrary to popular belief, MRI is not particularly expensive (it is perhaps double the cost of x-rays, but not much more), it is painless and non-invasive and has no known biological risks. Given that, it *should* be used frequently, or at least more frequently than expensive, painful, invasive and risky tests. The main downside of an MRI is the discovery of an incidental and irrelevant finding, one that will provoke unnecessary care or unnecessary worry. Simply: all patients for whom MRI is indicated should have one – but only them.

Because degenerative tears are so common, MRI should be avoided in a patient with a suspected degenerative meniscal tear – unless the test will affect management. At the least, weight-bearing x-rays should be obtained first to check for arthritis. Also, the patient should confirm interest in treatment should the test come back positive. In the setting of degenerative joint disease, a practitioner should have a high threshold for obtaining an MRI.

In the setting of an acute injury sustained by a young athlete, a practitioner should have a very low threshold for obtaining an MRI. Swelling and pain may limit the accuracy of the exam, and because it would be tragic to not detect a repairable injury before it progresses to an irreparable one (for example, a displaced but otherwise intact meniscal fragment that gets pulverized by the femoral condyle in its displaced position).

Meniscal tears are described by their configuration (Figure 7).

- A radial tear starts on the interior free margin of the meniscus and propagates peripherally,
- A horizontal cleavage tear lies within the meniscal tissue, parallel to the tibial plateau,
- A longitudinal tear is a top-to-bottom tear in the meniscus, the courses parallel to the capsule, perpendicular to the plateau.

Figure 7: A radial tear is highlighted in red; a horizontal cleavage tear is highlighted in blue; and a longitudinal tear is highlighted in green. (Modified drawing courtesy of Dr. Matt Skalski, Radiopaedia.org, rID: 55569.)

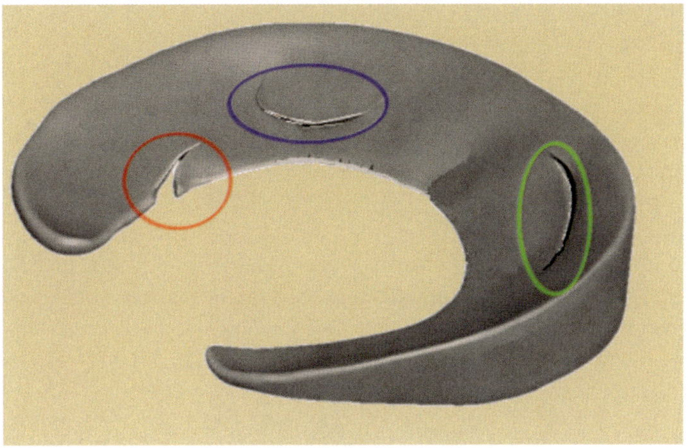

A bucket handle tear (Figure 8) is a specific form of a large longitudinal tear in which a large fragment is still tethered anteriorly and posteriorly, with the central piece flipped (like a bucket handle) into the intercondylar notch.

Figure 8: A bucket handle tear of the meniscus. The displaced fragment, tethered to the anterior and posterior aspects of the intact meniscus, is said to resemble the "bail handle" of a bucket—a loop that moves freely within two fixed mounts on the rim. (Drawing courtesy of Dr. Matt Skalski, Radiopaedia.org, rID: 55569. Photo courtesy Wikipedia)

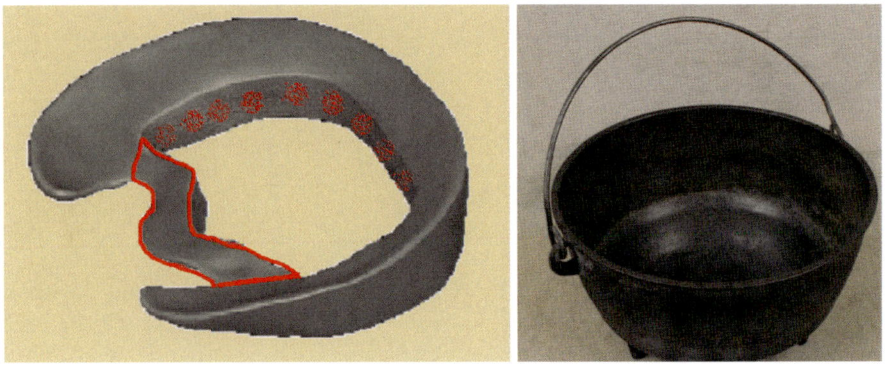

EPIDEMIOLOGY

Individuals who participate in sports are at the greatest risk for acute meniscal tears. Those who participate in sports where sudden change of movement is a critical component of the game (i.e. football, soccer, basketball) are at the most risk.

Degenerative tears are extremely common in older patients and often asymptomatic. The presence of a tear on MRI should not be assumed to be the source of symptoms.

DIFFERENTIAL DIAGNOSIS

Patients suspected to have an acute meniscus tear may have instead, or in addition, a collateral or cruciate sprain; an osteochondral injury; a loose body; or a disorder of the patello-femoral joint.

Patients suspected to have a chronic meniscus tear may have instead, or in addition, degenerative joint disease. Indeed, the presence of some degenerative joint disease can be assumed and the differential diagnosis pays attention to the relative contribution of each.

RED FLAGS

When evaluating the knee joint for a suspected meniscus tear, pay specific attention to detect associated injuries: a mechanism of injury that could tear the meniscus is a red flag for cruciate and collateral sprains, and vice versa.

A large effusion in young, active males may be a sign of gonorrhea. A detailed history is helpful here.

A locked knee suggests displacement of the meniscus into the notch, a so-called bucket handle tear.

A medial meniscal tear in a patient with a stable knee despite a known history of an anterior cruciate ligament deficiency is at high risk of developing symptomatic instability because of the meniscal tear. As such, a meniscal tear in this setting is a harbinger of impending problems and may provoke a need for anterior cruciate ligament treatment as well.

TREATMENT OPTIONS AND OUTCOMES

Displaced tears that prevent full motion should be considered for urgent surgery. The recommended procedure is an arthroscopy, with either a repair or removal of the tear, based on the intra-operative findings (Figures 9).

Figure 9: Arthroscopic view of a medial meniscus repair.

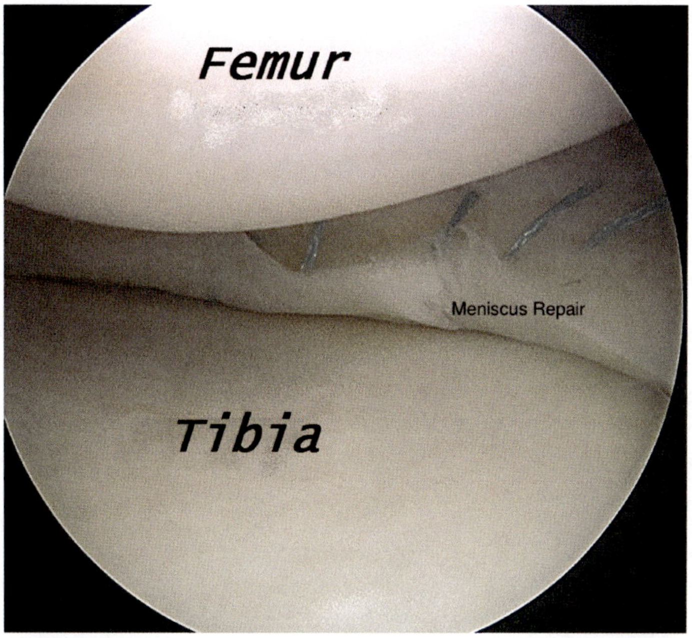

If the patient has full range of motion, urgent surgery is not indicated, unless imaging and the clinical scenario suggests a potentially repairable tear. (Tears in the outer 25% of the meniscus, in the red-red zone, have healing potential.) It is important to not miss the chance to treat a repairable tear while it is still repairable.

If the patient is planning surgery but deferring it (as may be done for a student waiting for an academic break in the calendar), protective bracing may be helpful.

Some meniscus tears, even acute ones, might become asymptomatic without surgery. Thus, it is reasonable for a patient to choose a trial of rest and anti-inflammatory medications, especially if the tear does not appear amenable to repair. The need for an arthroscopic meniscectomy will declare itself by a failure for symptoms to resolve.

In older patients, a course of physical therapy, working on strength and the maintenance of full motion, is reasonable. In one study from England, many patients on a waiting list for meniscal surgery cancelled their procedure before being called, as symptoms resolved spontaneously.

If the entire meniscus is torn and has to be removed, a meniscal transplant may be indicated in young patients with normal alignment and no arthritis.

The overall success rate of meniscal repair depends on the status of the ACL. If the ACL is intact, the meniscal tear will heal 60% of the time. If the ACL is injured, the meniscal tear will heal in 90% of cases if the ACL is reconstructed but in only 30% of cases if not. After removal of a large part of a meniscus, some patients have continued pain, likely due to the loss of the shock absorber effect. In rare cases, menisucs allograft transplantation can be performed, preparing a size-matched meniscus from a cadaver and securing it within the knee. Ideally, this operation is performed before any arthritic changes are found.

RISK FACTORS AND PREVENTION

The general risk factor for a meniscus tear is participation in sports, especially events that require high intensity shifting and change of direction.

A more focal risk factor is knee instability, especially a history of anterior cruciate ligament injury. With an ACL deficiency, the medial meniscus is called upon to help stabilize the knee, and is thus subjected to greater than normal forces.

There are no proven methods of prevention.

MISCELLANY

For many years, the menisci were thought to be vestigial, serving no specific function. Thus, surgeons routinely removed them. In 1948, Thomas John Fairbank published a paper, "Knee Joint Changes After Meniscectomy" in the *Journal of Bone and Joint Surgery* reporting that total meniscectomy produced squaring of the femoral condyles, peaking of the tibial spines ridging, and joint space narrowing. These are now known as Fairbank's changes.

The word meniscus comes from the Greek, mene, meaning moon. This is the same root that gives us the medical term "menstrual".

KEY TERMS

Medial and lateral menisci, meniscal tear, bucket handle tear

SKILLS

Identify locking, joint line tenderness and effusion on examination. Recognize meniscal tears on MRI. Recognize when MRI is indicated to detect meniscal tears.

CHAPTER 21.

CHONDRAL INJURIES OF THE KNEE

DESCRIPTION

Chondral injuries of the knee are lesions of the *articular* cartilage of the knee joint. (The colloquial expression "cartilage damage" might also include meniscal tears, which is an altogether separate category of disease.) Chondral injuries include both single focal defects and diffuse damage more characteristic of degenerative joint disease. Acute focal defects can accompany injuries such as an ACL tear and patellar dislocation. Articular cartilage damage can be seen with or without changes in the underlying bone. When bone pathology is absent, repair of the surface cartilage may be very helpful clinically, whereas when bone changes are present, the cartilage damage is merely the surface manifestation of the disease, and treating it alone is often futile.

STRUCTURE AND FUNCTION

The knee is a hinged synovial joint and consists of two articulations– the tibiofemoral and patellofemoral. The medial and lateral condyles of the femur rest on the tibial plateau to form the tibiofemoral articulation. The anterior aspect of the distal femur (trochlea) meets the patella to form the patellofemoral articulation. These joints are covered by articular cartilage.

In brief, articular (hyaline) cartilage decreases friction and distributes loads. The key to both properties is water: articular cartilage contains chondrocytes, proteoglycan and collagen molecules (almost all Type II), but at least 2/3rd of its mass is water. Articular cartilage has characteristic zones, in which the more superficial zone aspects have the collagen oriented parallel to the joint (for gliding) and the deep layer has its collagen oriented perpendicular to the joint (for compressibility). The deepest layer, the tidemark, is calcified and attaches to the subchondral bone (Figure 1). This organization distinguishes articular cartilage from the fibrocartilage that appears in some healing response. Fibrocartilage lacks this organization and thus lacks the normal mechanical properties and the durability of articular cartilage.

Figure 1: Schematic representation of articular cartilage resting on bone (B). The top layer (the lamina splendans) has horizontally aligned collagen molecules, to allow for sliding; the middle zone is oriented vertically, to resist compression. (Modified from https://www.intechopen.com/books/cartilage-tissue-engineering-and-regeneration-techniques/therapeutic-potential-of-articular-cartilage-regeneration-using-tissue-engineering-based-on-multipha)

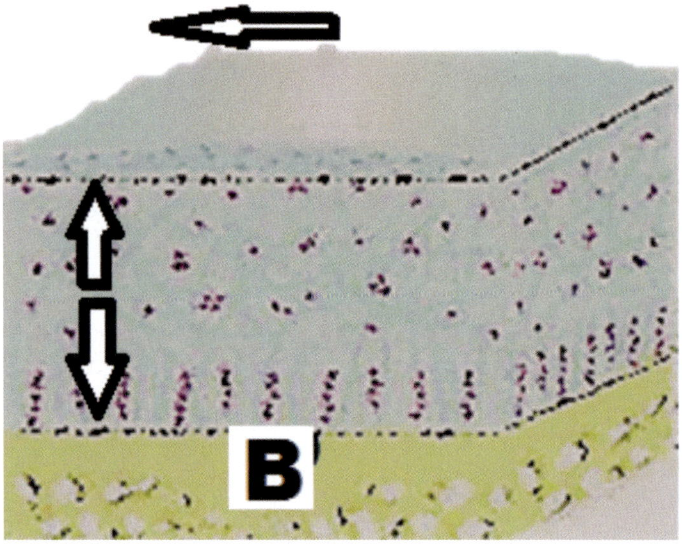

Another important biological principle regarding articular cartilage is that mild repetitive loading stimulates proteoglycan production whereas both immobilization and excessive repetitive loading leads to proteoglycan loss. That is to say, the health of the joint demands that the cartilage must be loaded within its physiological envelope of function: too much loading will cause damage, but too little loading will cause wasting.

The tibiofemoral articulation carries most of the body's weight across the knee (medial more than lateral). Because of leverage effects the patellofemoral joint is also exposed to high compressive forces. Both articulations are susceptible to articular cartilage injury.

PATIENT PRESENTATION

It is important to recall that patients do not present complaining of chondral injuries, per se. Rather they present complaining of a recent injury or subacute pain, and it is the examiner's task to determine whether a chondral lesion contributes to the presentation.

Chondral lesions commonly accompany injuries such as ACL tear and patellar dislocation. The cartilage is damaged by impact: in the case of an ACL tear, the tibia damages the lateral femoral condyle in a characteristic spot of contact (a so-called kissing lesion). Patellar dislocation can cause cartilage damage either as the bone goes out of place or when it is reduced (returns to the trochlea).

Defects can also be found incidentally on MRI or arthroscopy.

If there is no history of acute trauma, the pain usually is described as dull and aching. Patellofemoral lesions are usually associated with pain or discomfort after sitting for long periods of time. (This is known as the "theater sign".) Activity-related pain involves weight-bearing activities and are more common with tibiofemoral lesions. Other symptoms include effusion, catching, locking, and instability.

Other contributing factors may be noted on either history or physical exam, including prior patellar subluxation or dislocation, malalignment, or joint laxity due to ligamentous insufficiency.

The physical exam should assess patellar position and varus/valgus alignment. While sitting, assess quadriceps angle, tibial torsion, quadriceps atrophy (especially of the vastus medialis) and knee range of motion.

The supine exam should focus on effusion, decreased quadriceps or gastrocnemius flexibility, and patellar abnormalities. Tenderness to palpation over the joint line or directly over the femoral condyle would be expected with femoral condyle lesions. Pain with patellar compression would be expected with patellofemoral lesions.

OBJECTIVE EVIDENCE

X-rays are mainly used to rule out arthritis and assess for malalignment. Large osteochondral lesions, if present, will be apparent (Figure 2).

Figure 2: The arrow points at an osteochondral defect of the medial femoral condyle. (from https://radiopaedia.org/cases/osteochondral-defect-2?lang=us)

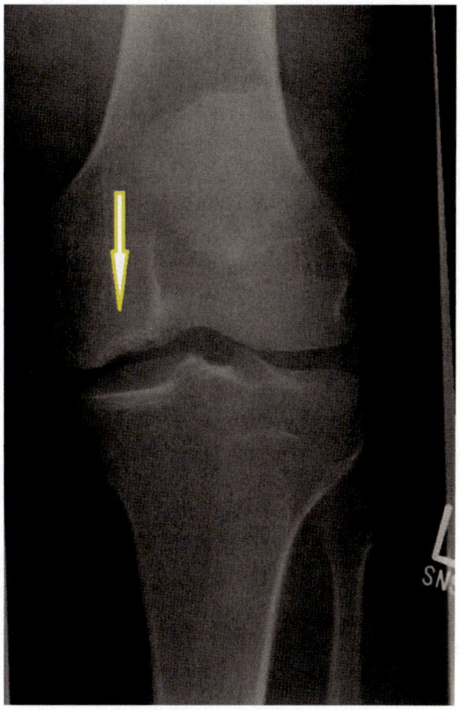

CT scanning is helpful when assessing patellar lesions, as it can more precisely measure the distance between the tibial tuberosity and the trochlear groove. Greater distances signify worse tracking of the patella and may prompt a need for surgical realignment.

MRI is the imaging of choice and most sensitive available for evaluating focal lesions (Figure 3). It also is the most essential for determining surgical vs. non-surgical management as it has the highest sensitivity and specificity for detecting osteochondral fragmentation.

Figure 3: The arrow points at an osteochondral defect of the medial femoral condyle. (from https://radiopaedia.org/articles/osteochondritis-dissecans?lang=us)

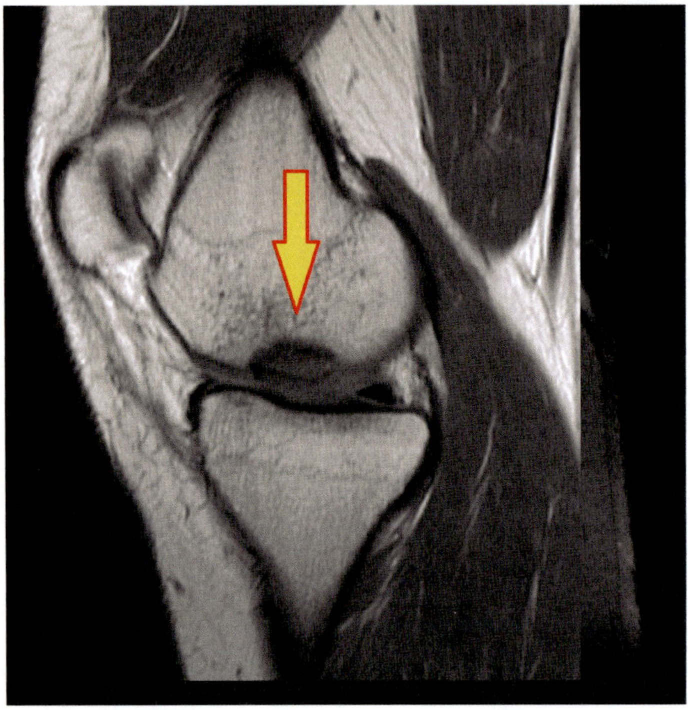

Lab findings are not usually helpful for evaluation of mechanical injuries such as chondral defects. However, inflammatory markers and disease-specific tests can be used to rule out inflammatory disease that may contribute to accelerated disease processes in the joints. Examples include systemic lupus erythematous and rheumatoid arthritis.

EPIDEMIOLOGY

Chondral injuries are more common in the adult and elderly population, likely a result of both degeneration and traumatic damage over time. About 10% of the population older than 40 years old have chondral defects. Traumatic knee injury can result in chondral defects in young patients.

DIFFERENTIAL DIAGNOSIS

Concomitant osteoarthritis and meniscus tears of the knee can present similarly to chondral lesions with pain, swelling, and mechanical issues such as catching.

An articular defect may also be due to osteochondritis dissecans. This is almost always present in the posterolateral aspect of the medial femoral condyle in skeletally immature patients. Recurrent effusions of the knee are commonly seen. This lesion is often amenable to treatment, and therefore it should not be missed. A child presenting with knee pain but without a significant history of trauma should raise appropriate clinical suspicion.

RED FLAGS

Chondral defects are usually associated with an effusion, and an effusion can of course suggest either septic or inflammatory arthritis. Aspiration and laboratory analysis of the fluid can be performed under the appropriate conditions to exclude these.

TREATMENT OPTIONS AND OUTCOMES

Treatment of a chondral lesion in the context of diffuse degenerative joint disease is dictated by the treatment needed for the arthritis.

For focal lesions, non-surgical management is the preferred initial treatment modality for most presenting cases and is the best route for those without significant symptoms. Common non-operative orthopedic management methods are used here, including activity modification, physical therapy, weight loss, exercise, NSAIDs and possibly corticosteroid injection.

Surgical management is considered in the young patient (<50 years old) who has attempted non-operative treatment with continued long-standing and functionally limiting symptoms, especially those related to a loose chondral fragment. Factors such as lesion size, depth, location, and status of the underlying chondral bone are all considered. At times, arthroscopy is needed to characterize the size and depth of the lesion (Figure 4).

Figure 4: The arrow points to a focal femoral condyle lesion seen at arthroscopy. (from https://ars.els-cdn.com/content/image/1-s2.0-S2212628719300490-gr3_lrg.jpg)

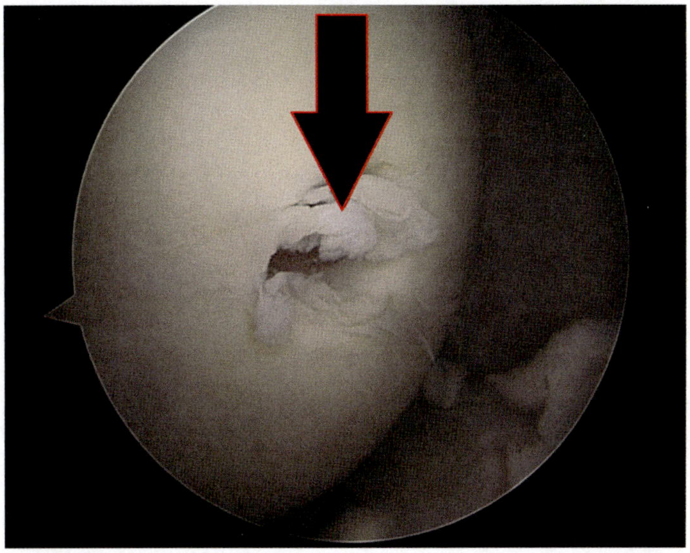

The classic surgical candidate is a young, active patient presenting with acute osteochondral fracture and full-thickness loss of cartilage. Strong contraindications to surgery include inflammatory disease and obesity. Relative contraindications include mechanical issues such as joint laxity, mal-alignment and ligamentous laxity.

The best form of surgical treatment leads to healing. Unfortunately, many articular lesions are not amenable to true healing. Fixation of a cartilage flap and drilling of the underlying bone is reliable only in patients with open growth plates, though this may be attempted in others.

Debridement, typically through arthroscopy, of course can clear debris and minimize mechanical symptoms, but given that the remaining articular cartilage is not normal, long-term positive results are hardly assured. Recall that the top layer is structurally and functionally different than the bottom layers, so damage to and loss of the superficial layer produces not only thinner articular cartilage but qualitatively worse articular cartilage: if there is surface abrasion, the top layer (the lamina splendans) is simply missing. This top layer helps protect the cartilage from damage, and its loss leaves it susceptible to further erosion.

There are a few techniques for filling defects: so-called marrow stimulation, in which fibrocartilage formation is induced; grafting; and chondrocyte implantation.

Marrow stimulation (also known as micro-fracture, abrasion chondroplasty and osteochondral drilling, depending on the specific method) aims to allow access of mesenchymal stem cells of the marrow into the articular defect to stimulate the formation of repair tissue, i.e. fibrocartilage. This technique is most effective in small lesions on the femur; it is less favored on the patella, in larger lesions, and in younger patients.

Grafting can be in the form of an autograft or an allograft. Osteochondral autografting fills a cartilage defect located in a critical area with plugs of normal autologous cartilage (with bone underneath) harvested from a less critical area. Ideally, the chondrocytes in the plug remain viable, and the bone heals into the subchondral bed in which it is placed (Figure 5).

Figure 5: The bone-and-cartilage plugs filling an articular defect are shown in this mini-arthrotomy. (from https://www.oatext.com/cartilage-damage-a-review-of-surgical-repair-options-and-outcomes.php)

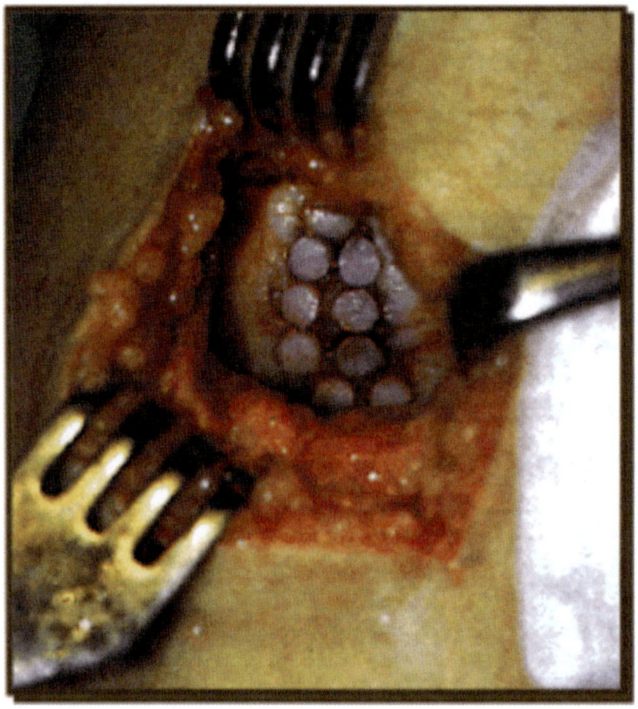

The "plug" technique is limited by the fact that articular cartilage will appear during early growth and development only in response to loadbearing. It is accordingly impossible to harvest cartilage from a non-weight-bearing part of a joint; at best one can hope to harvest from an area that is used sparingly. Accordingly, there may be some donor site morbidity when plugs are harvested. Also, the radius of curvature of the cartilage defect unlikely matches the radius of curvature of the harvested plug precisely.

Larger defects can be filled with cadaveric donor cartilage and bone. This technique of course brings with it the risk of infection, and chondrocyte viability may be lower.

Autologous chondrocyte implantation (ACI) attempts to foster regeneration of cartilage. The technique begins by harvesting a piece of native cartilage from the edge of the weight-bearing surface, usually from the intercondylar notch or periphery of the trochlea. Then, this is sent to a commercial laboratory where chondrocytes are isolated and encouraged to proliferate. This larger volume of cartilage cells are then re-implanted under a soft-tissue flap during a second procedure. This is the most expensive approach but does offer potential benefits that other operations lack.

If a defect arises from malalignment and uneven loading, then a realignment procedure may be indicted. In the patellofemoral joint, a tibial tubercle osteotomy may improve patellar tracking. In the tibiofemoral joint, a high tibial osteotomy or distal femoral osteotomy can help.

To date, the literature analyzing the long-term surgical outcomes of osteochondral defects is limited. A randomized controlled trial of adequate numbers of patients for the various operations (including a placebo), assessing not only short term function but long term avoidance of arthritis–the true measures of success–is highly infeasible.

RISK FACTORS AND PREVENTION

Risk factors include an unstable knee joint, malalignment and excessive repetitive activity. Addressing instability when it occurs should theoretically protect the joint surface, but it is unclear whether our methods of ligament reconstruction are sufficiently physiologic to truly protect the joint surface.

MISCELLANY

It is probably best to avoid the initials "OCD" to describe articular lesions, as these three letters may suggest both "**o**steo**c**hondral **d**efect" as well as "**o**steo**c**hondritis **d**issecans". There is some overlap between the two: however, there are important distinctions that should be preserved. Osteochondritis dissecans may be associated with a defect, but certainly not all defects represent osteochondritis dissecans. The treatment and prognosis of osteochondritis dissecans (especially in young patients) is altogether different than that of osteochondral defects in general.

KEY TERMS

Femoral condyle defect, patellofemoral defect, osteochondritis dissecans, microfracture, osteochondral autograft transfer, autologous chondrocyte implantation, transtibial-trochlear groove distance

SKILLS

Recognize and identify a chondral defect on imaging. Perform a physical exam to detect related instability or malalignment. Analyze imaging to characterize articular lesions.

CHAPTER 22.

COLLATERAL LIGAMENT INJURIES OF THE KNEE

DESCRIPTION

There are two collateral ligaments of the knee: the medial collateral ligament (MCL) and the lateral collateral ligament (LCL). Injuries of the MCL are much more common, owing to its exposure to damage from a blow to the outside of the knee, creating a so-called valgus force. Collateral ligament injuries can occur in isolation but also commonly occur in association with anterior cruciate ligament (ACL) and/or posterior cruciate ligament (PCL) injuries.

STRUCTURE AND FUNCTION

The knee has very little inherent bony stability: it has been described as two matchsticks held together by rubber bands. These "rubber bands" are the four main ligaments: the two cruciates, anterior and posterior; and the two collateral ligaments, medial and lateral (Figure 1 and Figure 2). These ligaments work in tandem to stabilize the knee. Other soft tissue structures, including the capsule, and the menisci also help provide stability. In general, the cruciates prevent anterior and posterior displacement of the tibia relative to the femur, and the collaterals provide side to side stability.

Figure 1: Schematic AP drawing of the medial (red) and lateral (green) collateral ligaments.

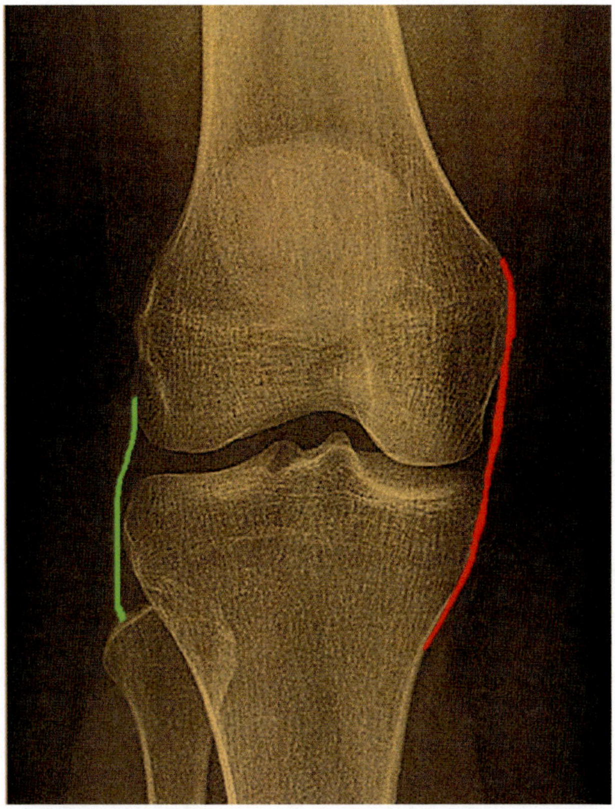

Figure 2: Schematic lateral drawing of the medial (red) and lateral (green) collateral ligaments.

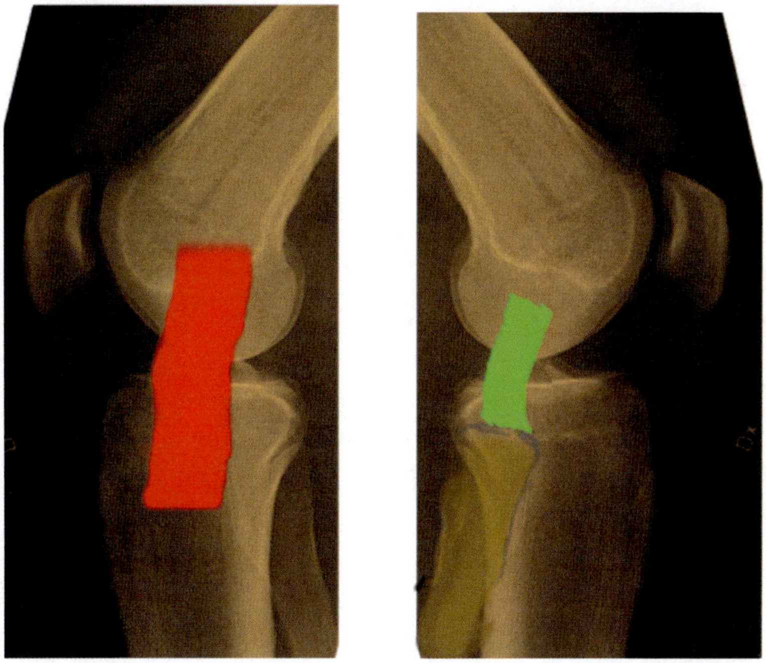

The main function of the medial collateral ligament, the MCL, is to resist valgus (knock-knee) deforming forces such as those generated by a blow to the outside of the knee with the foot planted.

The MCL consists of two bundles: a superficial bundle (the primary restraint), and a deep bundle, also known as the coronary ligaments (the secondary restraint). Additionally, the MCL works in concert with the ACL to resist axial rotation of the knee. The MCL originates from the medial femoral epicondyle and inserts on the medial proximal tibia extending down several centimeters. The deep bundle of the MCL attaches to the medial meniscus and is separated from the superficial bundle by a bursa. Posterior fibers of the deep MCL blend with the posteromedial capsule and posterior oblique ligaments. The MCL can accept up to 4000N of force without tearing.

The main function of the lateral collateral ligament, the LCL, is to resist varus displacement.

(A word on terminology: a valgus deformity is one in which the distal part is angled away from the midline; varus is in one in which the distal part angles towards the midline. At the knee, where these terms are most frequently used, it may be easier to simply memorize that valgus is "knock knee" and varus is "bow legged". These are shown in Figure 3.)

Figure 3: A normal alignment of the knee to the left; valgus in the middle; and varus to the right.

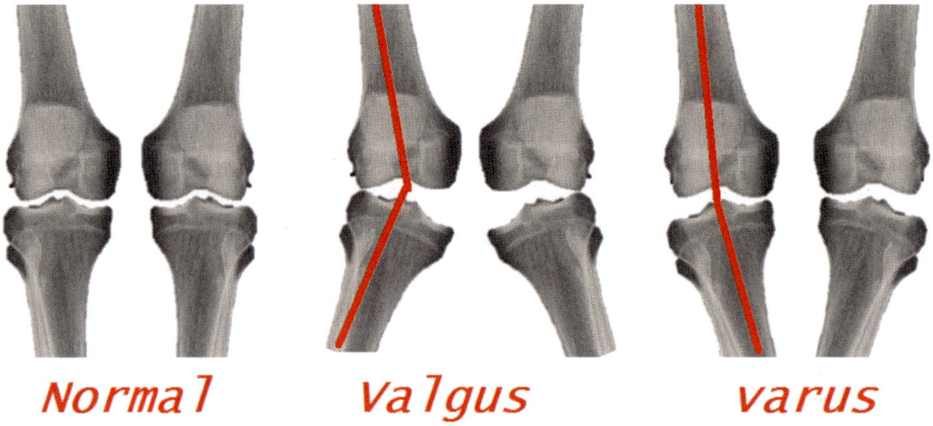

The LCL itself is much smaller than the medial collateral ligament. It originates from the lateral femoral epicondyle, posterior, superior, and superficial to the insertion of the popliteus. The LCL inserts on the fibula anterior to the popliteofibular ligament (PFL) on the fibula. The strength of the LCL has been measured at 750N vs. a varus stress. Stability on the lateral side is provided by the popliteus muscle and tendon as well as a collection of ligaments known as the "posterior lateral corner".

PATIENT PRESENTATION

Patients presenting with MCL Injuries usually describe being hit on the outside of their knee. There may be pain on the medial side where the ligament tears; there may be pain on the lateral side where the blow was sustained or where the femur and tibia contuse each other; and in the cases of a complete rupture of the ligament, there may be, surprisingly, little focal pain at all – just a general sense of difficulty ambulating and instability of the knee.

On physical exam, there can be tenderness to palpation along the medial joint line and more proximal. Ecchymosis may be present as well. A knee effusion may or may not be present. An effusion might be absent with a complete rupture of the medial collateral ligament as the torn tissue will let the joint fluid escape.

To isolate the medial collateral ligament on examination, stability is assessed with a valgus stress test at 30 degrees of knee flexion (Figure 4). In full extension, there is additional stability from the capsule that may mask a less severe MCL injury. If there is gapping in full extension, a combined injury is suspected.

Figure 4: The valgus stress test. The patient's knee is slightly flexed (off the edge of the table, as shown); a medially-directed force is applied to the knee by the examiner's hand closest to the patient's head, and a lateral force is applied the ankle.

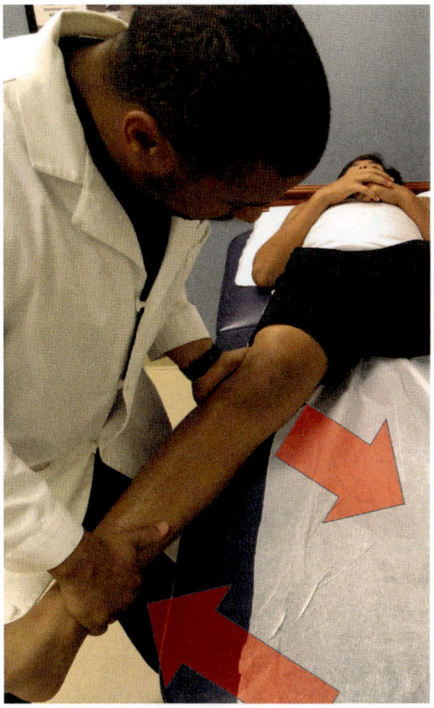

The grading of medial collateral ligament sprains is by the usual I, II and III classification, in which a Grade I sprain has little or no gapping on examination and a Grade III sprain, representing a complete tear, is defined by more than 10 mm of gapping or more than 10 degrees of increased valgus angulation. A Grade II sprain, characterized by plastic deformation of the ligament, will show some gapping but less than 10 mm.

An important aspect of the physical exam in these injuries is to evaluate the neurovascular structures of the knee. Evaluation of the saphenous nerve by checking sensation along the medial portion of the lower leg as well as palpation of the popliteal artery and distal vessels of the foot is necessary.

Injuries to the lateral collateral ligament are often in combination with other injuries, and the history and physical examination findings will be dominated by the other injuries. Stability against varus forces is assessed by analogous means, namely attempting to reproduce gapping with the knee in 30 degrees of flexion (Figure 5).

Figure 5: Varus stress test. The knee is slightly flexed and a lateral force is applied to the knee and a medial force on the ankle.

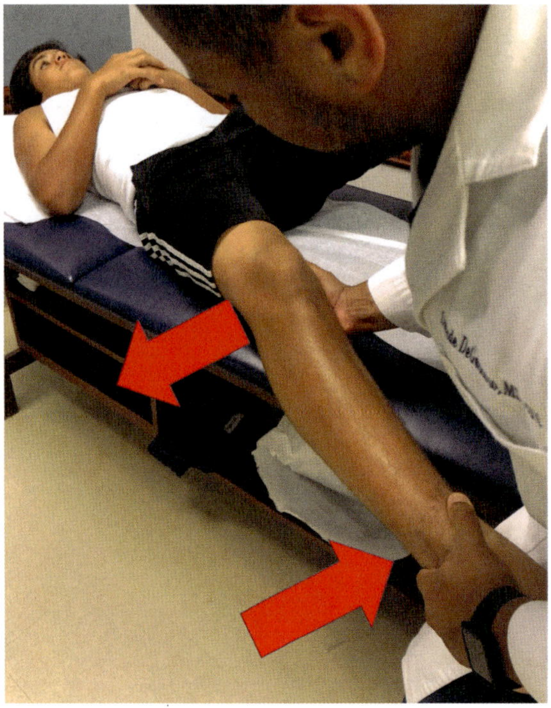

A thorough neurovascular exam should be performed to evaluate for injury to the common peroneal nerve when an LCL injury is suspected. A varus deforming force will apply traction to the nerve; because the nerve is tethered to the fibula, not much traction can be tolerated without injury.

High velocity mechanisms such as automobile accidents are apt to tear more than one ligament. A thorough physical exam is extremely important in these patients, including a thorough vascular exam. If there are multiple ligament injuries present, the knee joint may dislocate or subluxate. The incidence of an injury to the popliteal artery is approximately 50% in the setting of a knee dislocation.

After a thorough vascular exam, sensation should be assessed distinctly in the tibial, deep peroneal and superficial peroneal distributions. Motor examination should include flexor and extensor hallucis longus, tibialis anterior and gastrocnemius to establish baseline. The incidence of nerve injury ranges from 4.5% to 40%. The most commonly affected nerve is the common peroneal nerve, however isolated tibial nerve palsy has been reported.

Patients with some arthritis can present with a slight laxity on valgus stress testing with an intact medial collateral ligament. This is known as pseudo-laxity. The phenomenon is produced by the loss of articular cartilage causing narrowing of the medial joint space, which can then be corrected by the application of an external force.

OBJECTIVE EVIDENCE

For a patient presenting with a knee injury and possible ligamentous damage, radiographs with anteroposterior and lateral views are indicated.

Medial or lateral widening suggests possible ligament disruption. Considering that stress x-rays could worsen a partial ligament injury, they are not advised – especially since they are not apt to change the acute care management, and MRI can provide the same information, if not more.

For acute knee injuries, an MRI is extremely helpful. An MRI can provide information about severity (complete vs. partial rupture) and location (avulsion vs. mid-substance tear). Of course, an MRI will also pick up associated injuries. For chronic conditions, it may be helpful to employ an MRI if and only if the anticipated results of the test will dictate management (Figure 6).

Figure 6: An MRI showing a high grade MCL tear proximally (red arrow). The yellow arrow points to intact ligament distally. (Case courtesy of Dr. Tim Luijkx, Radiopaedia.org, rID: 48378)

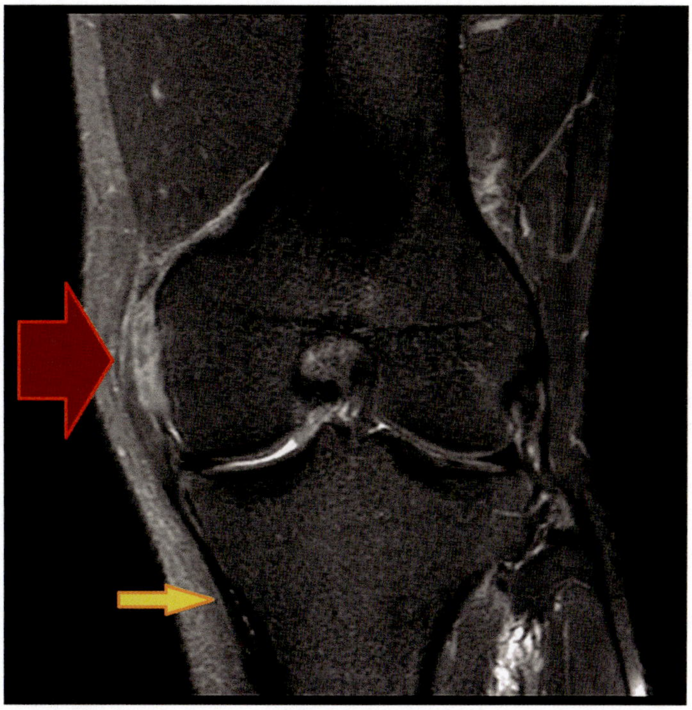

With chronic MCL injuries, calcification at the medial femoral insertion site may be seen. This is known as a Pellegrini-Stieda lesion (Figure 7).

Figure 7: A Pellegrini-Stieda lesion. A sliver of calcification is shown by the arrow. (Case courtesy of Dr. Charlie Chia-Tsong Hsu, Radiopaedia.org, rID: 18248)

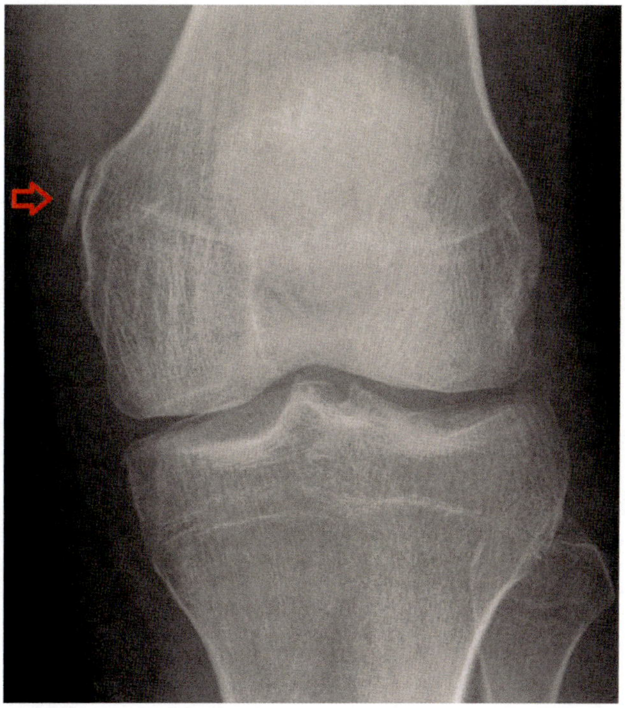

EPIDEMIOLOGY

Collateral ligament and multi-ligamentous injuries can occur in a variety of mechanisms thus leading to a very diverse patient population who suffer from these injuries. The most commonly injured ligament of the knee is the MCL.

Isolated injuries to the LCL are very rare. Injuries to the LCL are almost always found in combination with injuries to other ligaments, particularly posterolateral corner (PLC) injury.

Multi-ligamentous knee injuries most often occur as a result of high energy trauma, and perhaps due to gender differences in activities and risk seeking behaviors, are predominantly found in males. Low energy injuries that lead to multi-ligamentous knee injuries are almost exclusively limited to the obese population.

DIFFERENTIAL DIAGNOSIS

In addition to the collateral ligaments, the cruciates, the menisci, the extensor mechanism and the articular surfaces might be damaged by a sports injury. It is especially important here to remember the veterinary maxim 'a dog can have both lice and fleas', meaning the discovery of one injury does not signify the end of the examination as combined injuries are commonly seen.

In pediatric patients with open growth plates (physes), it is important to note that the MCL is typically more robust than the distal femoral physis, and thus, more resistant to injury. A suspected MCL tear in a patient with an open distal femoral growth plate, therefore, is more likely to have a physeal injury (fracture) than an MCL sprain and this may warrant a different treatment strategy.

RED FLAGS

Injury to more than one ligament suggests the possibility of injury to the popliteal artery or common peroneal nerve.

A loss of passive range of motion suggests interposed tissue (such as a piece of meniscus or articular cartilage). Another possible cause of blocked motion is "button holing" of the femoral condyle through the capsule. This finding is a clue to a more severe injury.

TREATMENT OPTIONS AND OUTCOMES

Because it is extra articular, the medial collateral ligament has good healing potential. Placing the patient in a brace can stabilize the knee and allow the ligament to heal at the appropriate length. Indeed, even if surgery is needed for other ligament injuries, it may be reasonable to allow the MCL to heal first.

Once some healing has taken place, physical therapy for quadriceps and hip adductor strengthening is indicated.

Operative repair may be considered for complete (Grade III) tears especially in the setting of multi-ligament knee injury. Another indication for surgery is if there is a displaced distal avulsion present–that is, if the MCL pulls off its tibial attachment. Surgery is needed because if the distal MCL retracts proximally, the pes anserine tendons will block healing.

For chronic injuries, or when there is loss of adequate tissue for repair, a reconstruction with either allograft or autograft is performed.

Treatment of LCL injuries is usually dictated by the presence of any associated injuries.

Most people with injuries to the medial collateral ligament will make a good functional recovery, but may require three months to get there.

Outcomes of LCL injuries are usually dictated by the response to treatment for the associated injuries.

RISK FACTORS

Risk factors for ligament injuries of the knee include participation in sports and obesity.

In high performance athletes who were unwilling to not play, the risk of MCL injuries (or worsening of an already present mild injury) may be mitigated by functional bracing.

MISCELLANY

Although the terms MCL, LCL, ACL and PCL are commonly used (and used above, as you see) all four sound sufficiently alike, especially to a lay person, that it may be better to avoid these shibboleths and sound out the words: “medial collateral”, “anterior cruciate”, etc..

KEY TERMS

medial collateral ligament, lateral collateral ligament, posterior-lateral corner

SKILLS

Detect MCL injury on exam. Detect associated injuries once collateral ligament injury is identified. Detect collateral ligament pathology on MRI.

CHAPTER 23.

CRUCIATE LIGAMENT DISORDERS

DESCRIPTION

The anterior cruciate ligament (ACL) and posterior cruciate ligament (PCL) connect the femur to the tibia and stabilize the knee joint, primarily in the sagittal plane (i.e., resisting anterior and posterior displacement, respectively). Of the two, it is the anterior cruciate ligament that is more frequently injured, either in isolation or with associated injuries to the meniscus, articular cartilage or collateral ligaments. Tears of the ACL typically occur when a person abruptly changes direction or decelerates with the foot planted. The less common PCL injury usually occurs when the tibia is forced poseriorly when the knee is flexed. The classic mechanism is an automobile accident in which the flexed knee strikes the dashboard after collision. The anterior cruciate ligament has very little healing potential, whereas the posterior cruciate ligament can occasionally repair itself.

STRUCTURE AND FUNCTION

The cruciate ligaments are named according to their attachment on the tibia: the anterior cruciate ligament courses from the posterior aspect of the intercondylar notch on the femur and inserts on the anterior tibial plateau. Similarly, the posterior cruciate ligament courses from a more anterior position in the notch to the posterior aspect of the proximal tibia. The term "cruciate" refers to the fact that these ligaments cross each other (Figures 1, 2 and 3).

Figure 1: The anterior (green) and posterior (red) cruciate ligament seen in the intrercondylar notch. The ACL courses from the lateral femur in a medial direction to insert on the tibia.

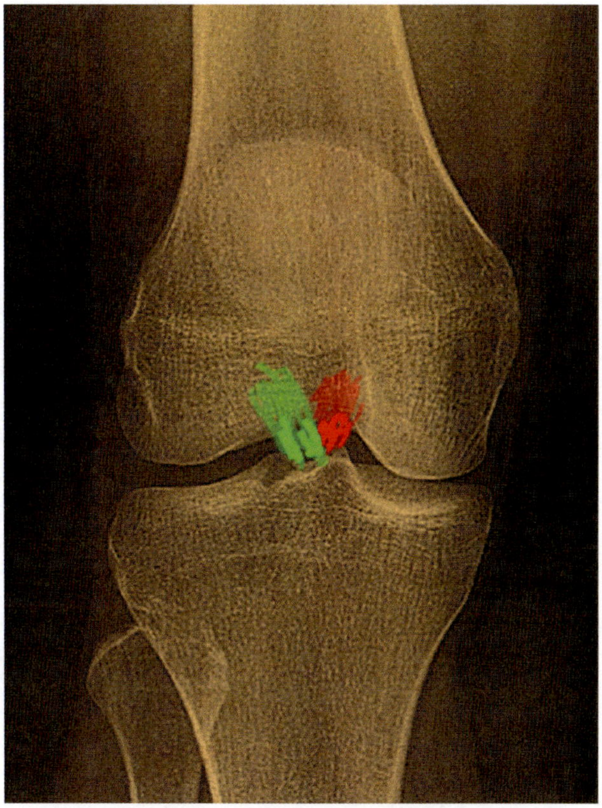

Figure 2: A lateral view showing the anterior (green) and posterior (red) cruciate ligaments. Note that ligaments are mostly vertical. This mostly-vertical orientation is suboptimal for resisting anterior/posterior translation but allows the knee to flex and extend more freely than a purely horizontal orientation would allow. Note also that the ACL inserts on the top of the tibia (the plateau) whereas the PCL inserts about 1 cm below the joint line.

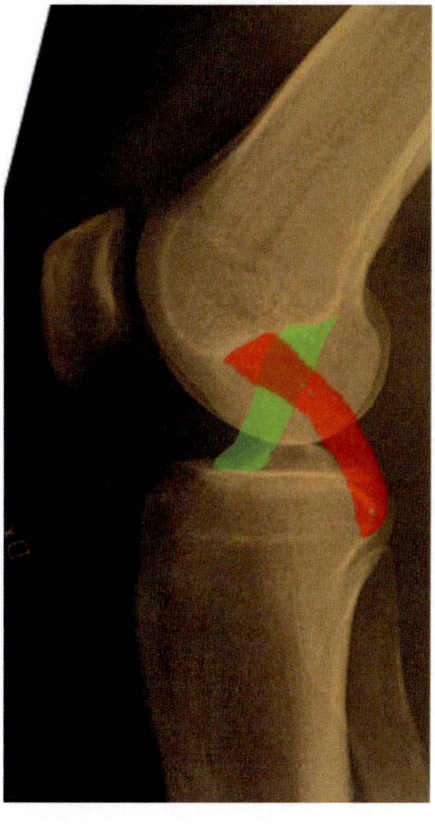

Figure 3: An MRI sagittal slice within the notch showing the anterior cruciate (green) and a small piece of the posterior cruciate (red). Because the ACL courses lateral (femur) to medial (tibia) and the PCL medial to lateral, it is rare to see both ligaments simultaneously on one single MRI image (from https://radiopaedia.org/images/20228493)

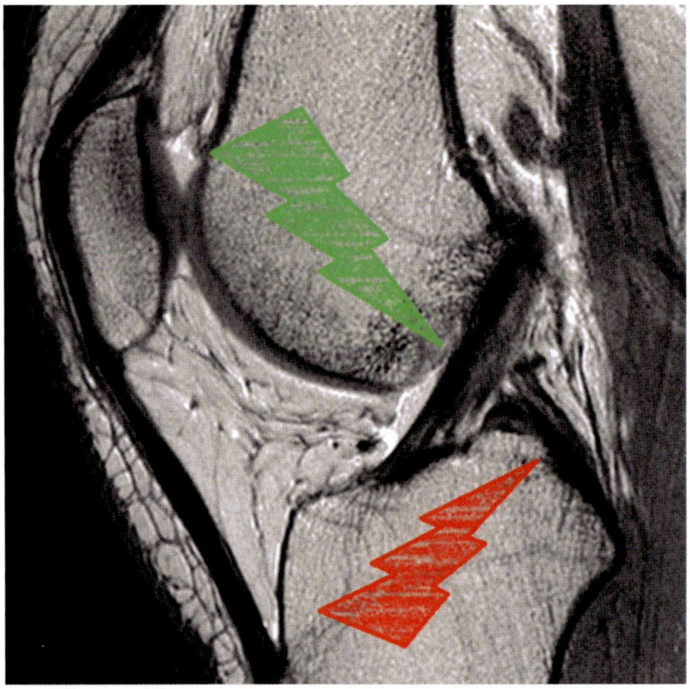

The ACL has been described having two bundles: the anteromedial bundle and the posterolateral bundle. This distinction is somewhat arbitrary as the boundary between bundles is not stark. A better way to think about it, perhaps, is that there are different regions of the ligament, with the anteromedial aspect more taut in flexion and the posterolateral aspect more taut during extension.

Injury to the ACL is usually caused by excessive force moving the tibia anterior relative to the femur, sometimes in combination with internal rotation of the tibia at the knee. This rotation increases the distance between the origin and insertion of the ligament, such that the ligament is under greater tension for a given degree of anterior displacement.

Varus or valgus (clipping) forces at the knee can also injure the ACL but only after the affected collateral ligament is injured first.

So-called cutting maneuvers (rapid changes in direction while running) are very common mechanisms for ACL injuries. When the foot is planted the tibia is anchored in space, whereas the body's center of gravity may pull the femur in a different direction.

Mechanoreceptor nerve fibers are found within the ACL and provide proprioception. Thus, an injury can create a sense of instability not only because of the loss of passive restraint but because of the loss of proprioception.

The PCL also lies within the intercondylar notch. It originates from the inner aspect of the medial femoral condyle and attaches to the posterior aspect of the proximal tibia, slightly below the joint line.

Like the ACL, the PCL also has two bundles, called the anterolateral bundle and the posteromedial bundle. The anterolateral bundle is tightest in knee flexion and prevents posterior translation of the tibia relative to the femur. The posteromedial bundle is tightest in extension of the knee and prevents hyperextension of the knee.

A posterior-directed force that pushes the tibia backwards while the knee is flexed can tear the PCL. Alternatively, a force that causes sufficient hyperextension of the knee can also cause a PCL injury, but this is less commonly seen.

The PCL is at least 25% stronger than the ACL, being able to resist forces up to 3000 N.

PATIENT PRESENTATION

Patients with a torn ACL will typically present with immediate swelling and pain.

Patients will commonly report hearing a popping sound or perceiving a popping sensation at the time of the injury.

The classic mechanism of injury for an ACL tear is a non-contact injury after a sudden pivot with the leg planted – think of a skier whose ski is fixed on the snow and twists his or her torso.

The knee may fill with blood (forming a so-called hemarthrosis). This fluid collection may make motion painful, but also may stabilize the knee. This false stability is enough to mask the tear on examination.

The most sensitive physical exam maneuver for detecting a torn ACL is the Lachman test, where the femur is stabilized while the tibia is pulled forward (Figure 4). A positive test is signified by excessive forward translation without a firm endpoint, indicating disruption to the ACL. Because the Lachman test is assessed by the perceived firmness of the endpoint – an intact ACL will stop anterior translation more suddenly – experienced examiners will perform the test more accurately.

Figure 4: Lachman Test: The examiner stands next to the supine patient and grasps the lateral thigh just above the knee with the upper (contralateral) hand to exert resistance (blue line). The examiner holds the tibia medially with the lower (ipsilateral) hand, flexes the knee to 30 degrees and then applies a jerking force to the tibia, in an attempt to subluxate it in an anterior direction (blue arrow). As shown, this will place tension on the ACL (drawn in red).

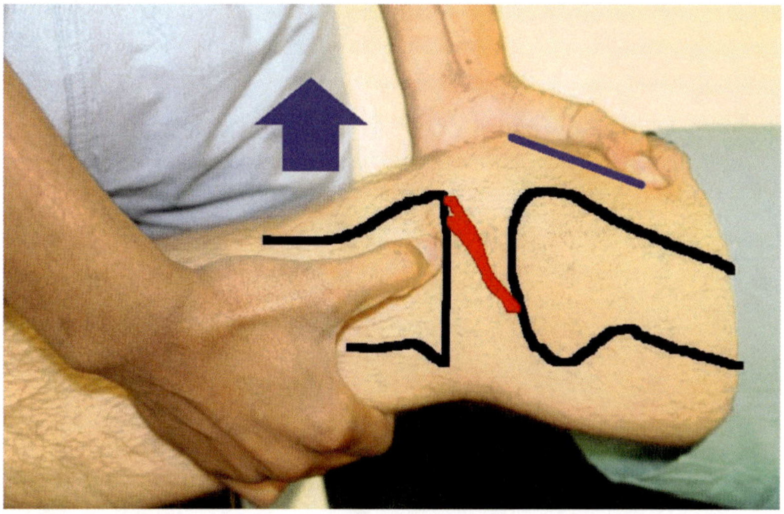

The anterior drawer test (simply assessing whether there is an abnormal amount of anterior displacement when a force is applied to the flexed knee) is another physical exam maneuver that is similar to the Lachman test but is less accurate. That is because a varying degree of anterior translation is normal, and whether what the examiner is perceiving represents an abnormal amount may be difficult to tell.

Another specific test to assess for ACL instability is the pivot shift test. This test is a diagnostic maneuver that moves the tibia in and out of its normal anatomical position, if and only if the ACL is damaged. The test is performed with the examiner grasping the leg and holding the knee in extension (with a slight internal rotation torque to the tibia). In this position, the tibia will subluxate anteriorly relative to the femur if the ACL is torn. The knee is then flexed. In flexion, the knee is in its normal position, even if the ACL is torn. Thus, if the knee is noted to clunk back into position during flexion, the test is positive (for a torn ACL). This test may be difficult to perform in the apprehensive patient, but is a critical component of the physical examination when performed under anesthesia.

Tests for ACL tears can be falsely negative if there is a displaced fragment of either bone or cartilage in the knee or if the hamstrings are resisting the examiner. Also, as noted, the fluid in the knee may stabilize it somewhat and therefore if there is a tense effusion the Lachman test may be falsely negative as well.

It may be diagnostically and therapeutically helpful to aspirate the knee. Removing the volume of fluid will make the patient more comfortable. Also, merely assessing the color of the fluid helps with diagnosis (red, meaning blood, signifies a clinically important injury in approximately 90% of cases). In addition, by draining the knee, a more reliable physical examination can be performed.

Patients with chronic deficiency of the anterior cruciate ligament present with a "trick knee", that is a sense of instability. They may also present with the stigmata of arthritis, as the loss of the ACL leads to abnormal biomechanics which in turn can cause articular damage.

The classic presentation of a patient with a PCL injury is generalized knee pain, a limp, and mild to moderate knee swelling.

Patients with injuries to the PCL do not typically describe a popping sensation, but they may report a direct blow to the knee.

The most accurate physical exam maneuver for PCL tears is the posterior drawer test, where the knee is flexed at 90 degrees and a posterior force is applied to the anterior proximal tibia, driving it backwards. A positive sign is excessive posterior translation of the tibia relative to the femur, as compared to the uninjured side and the lack of a firm endpoint.

Patients with chronic PCL deficiency do not complain of instability but rather anterior knee pain. That is because patients have learned to stabilize their knee by "holding on" to their tibia with active quadriceps force. This quadriceps force loads the patellofemoral joint causing articular degeneration.

OBJECTIVE EVIDENCE

While x-rays can and should be obtained to rule out concomitant fracture or avulsion injury to the bones of the knee (i.e., Segond fracture – a fleck of bone off the anterolateral tibia that is pathognomonic for ACL injury), the gold standard imaging modality for definitive diagnosis of both ACL and PCL injuries is an MRI of the knee (Figure 5).

Figure 5: An MRI showing a torn ACL (red arrow) (from https://radiopaedia.org/articles/anterior-cruciate-ligament-tear)

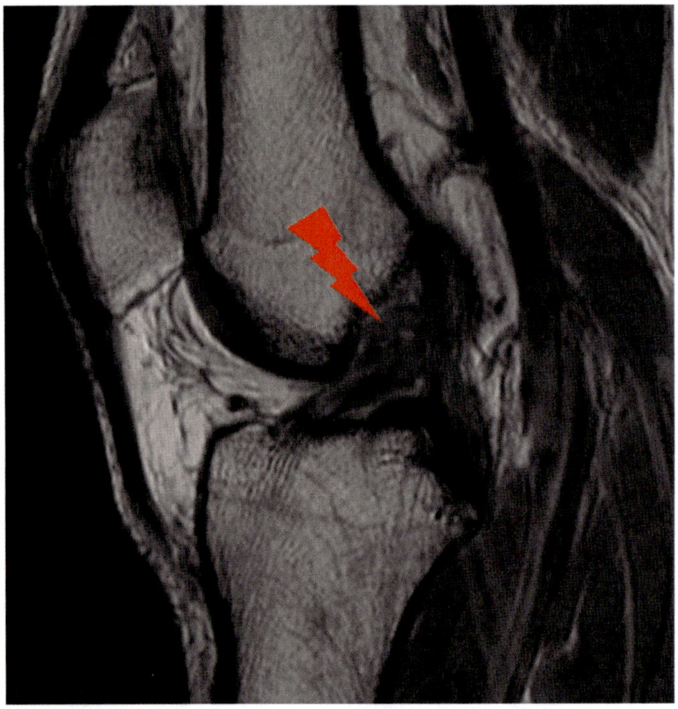

On sagittal view, absence or discontinuity of ACL fibers would indicate an ACL injury.

The classic finding for an ACL tear on MRI is a so-called kissing contusion on both the tibia and femur: this is a bone bruise caused by the impact of the lateral tibial plateau into the middle of the femoral condyle, a region known as the sulcus terminalis.

EPIDEMIOLOGY

ACL injury is common in athletes, especially in the high school age group. Female athletes are particularly prone to ACL injury. However, ACL injury is still common in college and professional athletes, as well as the general population. The estimated incidence of ACL injuries per year is about 200,000 in the United States. Approximately half of all ACL tears are isolated injuries; the other half are associated with either damage to the meniscus or collateral ligaments.

PCL injuries are less common, owing to the ligament's greater strength but also because pivoting while running is not apt to tear it. The most common mechanism of PCL injury involves motor vehicle accidents, with contact from the dashboard against the flexed knee pushing the tibia in a posterior direction.

DIFFERENTIAL DIAGNOSIS

In the acute setting, the goal is to identify all of the injured structures. Concomitant injuries are common.

Assuming radiographs do not show a fracture, the other structures that might be injured include the collateral ligaments, the menisci and the articular surfaces.

Patella dislocations may occur with a history that suggest a cruciate ligament injury: namely, a twisting mechanism, a sense of a "pop" and bleeding into the knee.

The PCL in particular is usually associated with other ligamentous injury, especially injuries to the posterolateral corner of the knee, which tends to make it relatively more difficult to diagnose compared to ACL injury.

Bony contusions, fractures, and knee dislocation are also generally included in the differential diagnosis for PCL injuries.

RED FLAGS

A patient's inability to fully extend the knee may be due to a displaced tear of the meniscus. This requires urgent arthroscopic surgery not only to remove the mechanical block and restore the range-of-motion of the knee but to possibly preserve the tissue for repair.

A young male patient may present with both an effusion and a history of knee pain after playing sports but the two may not be related. Rather, the joint fluid in this case may actually be caused by gonorrhea. This can be assessed by a short question about urethral symptoms.

TREATMENT OPTIONS AND OUTCOMES

Patients with less severe ACL injury or willingness to modify their activities may be successfully treated with physical therapy and some degree of immobilization (e.g. use of a brace while playing sports).

There is a school of thought (more so in Europe than in the United States) that perhaps all patients should be treated non-operatively at first, as many will do fine with therapy alone. The downside to this approach is that those patients who are unstable enough to ultimately need surgery often inflict greater damage on the knee in the interval between the initial injury and the surgical treatment.

Younger patients, athletes, and those with severe instability of the knee are more likely to require operative reconstruction in order to return to their desired activity level. ACL tears should be evaluated by an orthopedic surgeon to determine if surgery is indicated.

The first consideration when contemplating surgical repair of PCL injuries is the degree of injury. If not torn completely, the PCL has particularly high potential to heal with immobilization and then therapy. These exercises can assist with stability of the knee, particularly by strengthening the quadriceps muscles (which have an anterior-directed vector in their normal action).

PCL surgery is most commonly indicated when there is another injury (e.g., the posterior-lateral corner ligaments) when patients continue to have persistent feelings of posterior tibial instability or, more commonly, they develop *anterior* knee pain. That pain reflects overuse of the quadriceps to stabilize the knee, which then produces overload to the patellofemoral joint.

In both ACL and PCL injury, surgical repair involves replacement of the injured ligament with a graft (Figure 6). This may be from the patient's own patellar or hamstring tendons or from a cadaver. The damaged ligament itself is removed and discarded. The repair is typically done arthroscopically.

Figure 6: Arthroscopic view of ACL reconstruction graft (arrow) in the notch. The white fibers of the PCL are seen to the right of the graft ("P") (from commons.wikimedia.org/wiki/File:Anterior_cruciate_ligament_repair_2.jpg)

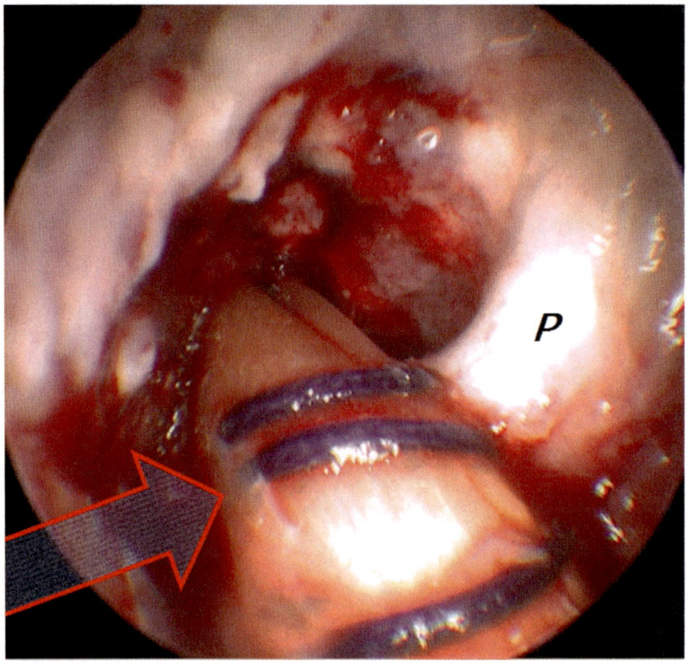

Autografts are generally favored over allografts in patients 25 years old or younger, given the lower rate of re-tears as compared to allografts in this population.

The surgery for ACL and PCL reconstruction typically involves creating tunnels in the bone of the tibia and femur through which the grafted tendon will be inserted and fixed. These are then fixed into the tunnels, typically with screws. Other techniques can be used as well, but they all generally involve fixation of the graft on either end onto the bone of the femur and tibia.

Both ACL and PCL surgical repairs require postoperative rehabilitation. Rehabilitation exercises focus on regaining normal range of motion and strengthening the quadriceps and hamstring muscles. Care must be taken not to overload or overstress the graft during the initial phases of healing.

The outcomes for ACL reconstruction are generally very good at least in the medium term. In the past, ACL tears in particular would end careers for professional athletes, but improvements in surgical reconstruction have allowed athletes to essentially regain full functional stability. It is common to see patients return to their high-level performance. The long term risk of arthritis does loom, as even the best surgical reconstruction is not as good the native ligament, and the articular surface may have been irreparably damaged by the impact at the time of injury.

The outcomes of PCL reconstruction are typically very good to excellent, but because the surgery is reserved for only severe injuries, usually, the knee is not perfect post-operatively.

With both ACL and PCL injuries, outcomes are worse if there is a concomitant articular or meniscal injury.

RISK FACTORS AND PREVENTION

For ACL injury, risk factors include high school age, female gender, and playing soccer or basketball. For PCL injury, athletes such as American football linemen may be at increased risk.

Prevention of either injury relies upon strengthening of the muscles that stabilize the knee joint and promote endurance. It is not uncommon to see ACL tears later in the day on the ski slopes, which may reflect the loss of hamstring stabilization due to muscle fatigue. That is, if the hamstrings are tired and weak, they may not be able to hold on to the tibia, which then exposes the ACL to greater forces. Teaching proper landing technique may also reduce risk of ACL injury.

KEY TERMS

Arthroscopy, anterior cruciate ligament, posterior cruciate ligament, knee, tibial plateau

SKILLS

Examination of cruciate ligament injuries to the knee.

CHAPTER 24.

ACHILLES TENDON DISORDERS

DESCRIPTION

The Achilles tendon is subject to high forces with each step and therefore subject to wear-and-tear damage. There are many pathological conditions that affect the Achilles tendon, but the most common chronic conditions are tendonitis and bursitis. The most common acute condition is an Achilles rupture (often superimposed on wear-and-tear).

STRUCTURE AND FUNCTION

The Achilles tendon is the largest and strongest tendon in the human body. It attaches the posterior calf muscles (the gastrocnemius and soleus) to the calcaneus.

Figure 1: The Insertion of the Achilles Tendon (red arrow)

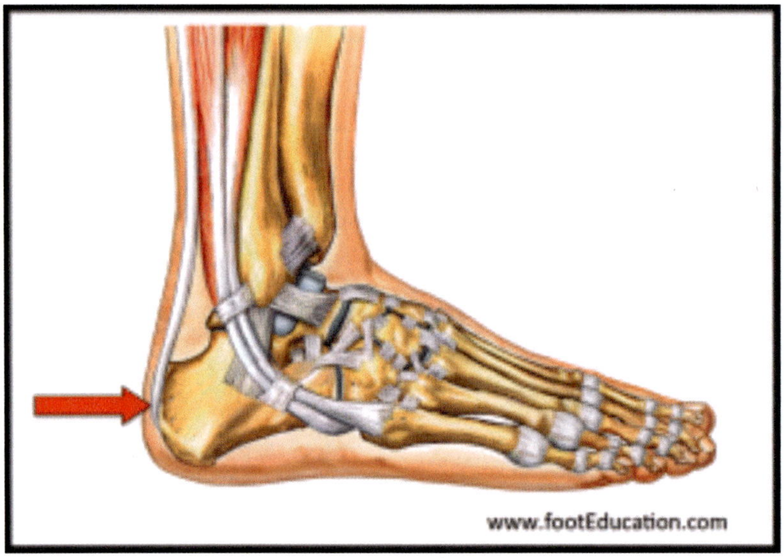

The posterior calf muscles both actively plantar flex the ankle and resist passive dorsiflexion during walking, jumping, and running. Note that when the person places the ball of his or her foot on the ground during gait, body weight and momentum will force the ankle into dorsiflexion. Resisting this motion, and in turn decelerating the landing of the heel, is powered by the posterior calf muscles. Forces up to 3 times body weight may be applied to the tendon when this happens while walking; even greater forces are applied while jumping and running. The Achilles tendon inserts into the posterior surface of the calcaneus. The insertion begins about halfway between the plantar and superior surface of the calcaneus (Figure 1).

A bursa lies between the tendon and calcaneus above the insertion point: the so-called retrocalcaneal bursa. Another bursa lies posterior to the tendon between the tendon and skin, namely, the subcutaneous calcaneal bursa. A bursa is a fluid-filled sac (the word shares its origin with the English word "purse") that normally exists between tendons and bone in places where the bone surface may be prominent; this allows the tendon to glide more easily. In the healthy state, the bursa is only a few cells thick, and the bursa is filled with only a small amount of lubricating fluid. However, when irritated, a bursa can become markedly thickened and filled with larger amounts of fluid. This condition is known as bursitis.

PATIENT PRESENTATION

Achilles tendonitis is a chronic condition characterized by pain and swelling in the Achilles tendon.

Symptoms of tendonitis are produced by swelling and inflammation of the tissue that surrounds the Achilles tendon – the paratendon. As such, the condition may be more appropriately described as an Achilles tenosynovitis (inflammation of the lining surrounding the Achilles tendon). Inflammation of the tendon can be caused either by direct pressure from shoewear or more commonly, as part of the healing response to over-use and micro-trauma.

There are two types of Achilles tendonitis: non-insertional tendonitis and insertional tendonitis.

Achilles Tendonitis (Non-Insertional)

In classic non-insertional (or mid-substance) Achilles tendonitis, the pathology is typically located 2 to 6 cm proximal to the insertion of the Achilles tendon to the calcaneus.

Non-insertional Achilles tendonitis is often associated with a history of increased activity level (e.g., starting a new training regimen or attempting to resume a normal activity level after an injury and enforced immobilization).

Figure 2: Location of Symptoms: Non-insertional Achilles (Left) and Insertional Achilles (right)

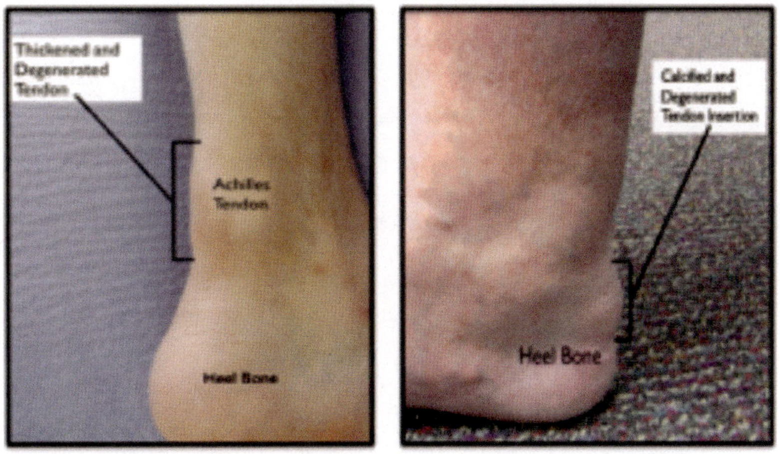

A patient presenting with non-insertional Achilles tendonitis (Figure 2 left) will often describe pain and tenderness 2-6 cm from the insertion of the tendon into the calcaneus. The patient will often describe an increase in activity, such as starting a new training regimen or attempting to resume a normal activity level after an injury to another part of the foot or ankle.

Physical Examination will usually reveal swelling and tenderness around the Achilles tendon. There is often an associated tight calf muscle (equinus contracture). The location of the pain can help differentiate this from insertional tendonitis (Figure 2 right) which presents with pain more distally.

Insertional Achilles Tendonitis

In so-called "insertional" Achilles tendonitis, the pathology is located at the insertion of the Achilles tendon to the calcaneus (Figure 2, right). Insertional Achilles tendonitis is a product of wear and tear at the attachment ("insertion") of the tendon onto the calcaneus. This degeneration incites an inflammatory response and produces pain at the back of the heel. Eventually, the inflamed Achilles tendon may become calcified, forming bone-like fragments in the tendon.

The pathology associated with insertional Achilles tendonitis includes the "terrible triad" (Figure 3):

1. Degeneration of the Achilles tendon near the insertion site,
2. An inflamed retrocalcaneal bursitis, and
3. A Haglund's deformity (a prominent bony lump on the heel).

Figure 3: Location of pain in patients with the "Terrible Triad": insertional Achilles tendonitis, retrocalcaneal bursitis, and a prominent bony lump on the heel (known as a Haglund's deformity).

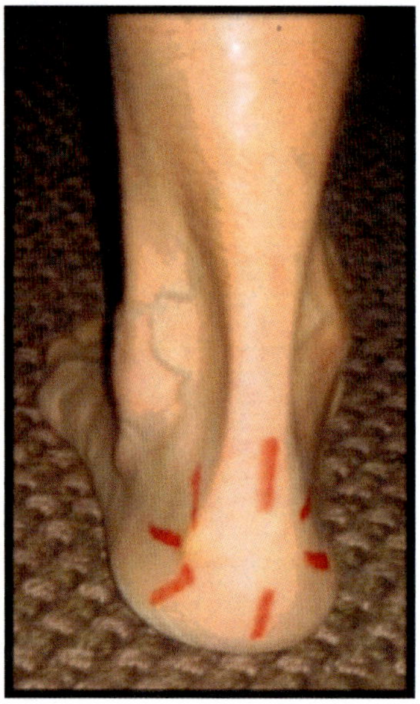

A Haglund's deformity is a bony prominence associated with the upper part of the calcaneus (Figure 4). This is sometimes called a "pump bump." This prominent bone tends to form gradually over many years, and can eventually cause irritation by disrupting nearby structures, including the retrocalcaneal bursa and the Achilles tendon. The bony prominence also creates discomfort by rubbing up against the back of footwear, the so-called "heel counter" of the shoe.

Figure 4: Haglund's Deformity. An x-ray showing both a Haglund's deformity (red arrow) as well as calcification of the Achilles tendon insertion (white arrow)

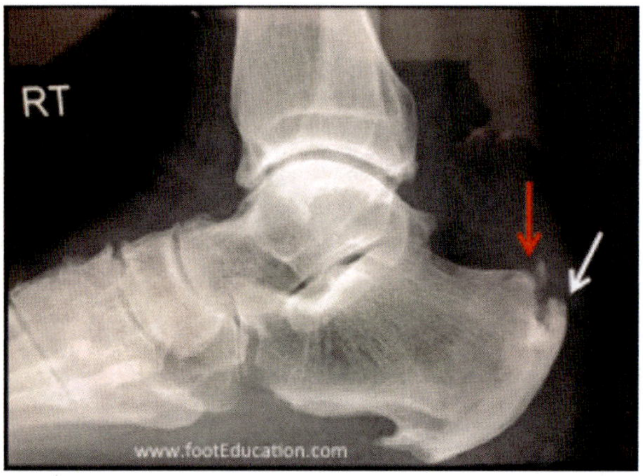

When a Haglund's deformity is present, the retrocalcaneal bursa can become inflamed. This inflammation can result in exquisite tenderness along the posterior aspect of the heel.

OBJECTIVE EVIDENCE

X-rays will usually be negative in cases of non-insertional Achilles tendonitis, unless there is calcification of the Achilles tendon. (Calcification is relatively rare except in older patients.) Cases of insertional Achilles tendonitis may reveal a calcaneal spur on x-ray.

An MRI can give a detailed view of the soft tissue (Figure 5). However, this test is not routinely indicated in the initial assessment of Achilles tendonitis.

Ultrasound is usually less expensive than an MRI, but may not be available in all settings. Further, use of ultrasound may be limited by the examiner's lack of skill or experience.

Figure 5: MRI of Achilles Tendonitis (non-insertional) Swelling associated with non-insertional Achilles tendonitis as seen on MRI. The tendon is shown in continuity but is abnormally thickened.

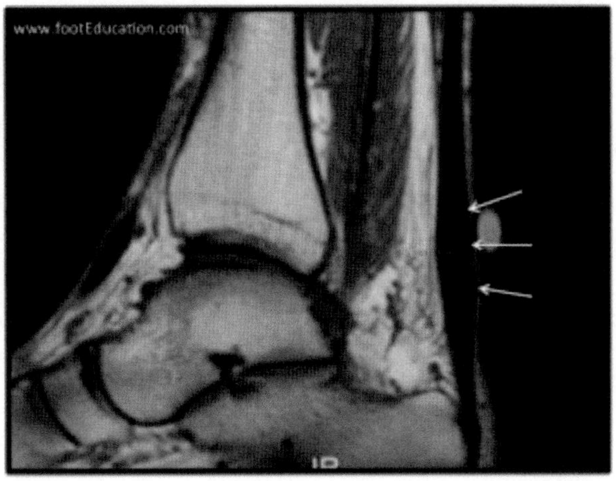

EPIDEMIOLOGY

Insertional Achilles tendonitis with its associated "terrible triad" of heel pain typically occurs in middle-aged individuals who are overweight, though a variant of this condition is also seen in young, active runners. The exact incidence of this bimodal distribution has not been recorded.

Non-Insertional Achilles tendonitis is often associated with an increase in activity level/overuse and tends to occur in patients in their 30s and 40s. According to Jarvinen et al., the reported annual incidence of Achilles tendonitis is between 7-9% in top-level runners (PMID: 15922917).

DIFFERENTIAL DIAGNOSIS

There are four common causes for pain near the back of the heel:

1. non-insertional Achilles tendonitis,
2. insertional Achilles tendonitis (with or without bursitis),
3. paratendonitis (inflammation of the sheath surrounding the Achilles tendon, rather than of the tendon itself), and
4. Achilles tendon rupture.

The Thompson test will identify an Achilles tendon rupture. The precise location of the pain should distinguish non-insertional Achilles tendonitis vs insertional Achilles tendonitis.

RED FLAGS

Although corticosteroid injections in and around the Achilles can be helpful in the short-term managing symptoms they weaken the tendon and predispose to tearing. Be alert for patients that have had corticosteroid injections in this area.

Patients with inflammatory arthropathies may also get inflammation in the lining around their Achilles. If a patient has other joints that are painful or swollen, especially if they are of recent onset, an inflammatory etiology should be ruled out.

TREATMENT OPTIONS AND OUTCOMES

Non-operative Treatment of Achilles Tendonitis

Most patients with Achilles tendonitis can have their symptoms treated effectively without surgery. Insertional Achilles tendonitis can be more recalcitrant to treatment than non-insertional Achilles tendonitis. An initial period of relative rest to allow the symptoms to settle is often beneficial. This is followed by a gradual return to normal activities incorporating the following non-operative treatment elements:

1. Activity modification,
2. Shoewear modification (a heel lift will unload the tendon),
3. Weight Loss (if applicable),
4. Anti-inflammatory medication (if not contra-indicated) and,
5. A rehabilitation program including specific stretching and strengthening exercises.

Stretching the gastrocnemius (outer calf muscle) with the knee straight (Figure 6) is an important component of non-operative treatment. A tight calf muscle will increase the force going through the Achilles tendon and predispose the tendon to micro-tearing.

A graduated eccentric loading program (strengthening the calf muscle while it is lengthening) is an important component of non-operative treatment for non-insertional Achilles tendonitis (Figure 7). However, it may be too aggressive for patients with insertional Achilles tendonitis.

Using a heel lift reduces the "stretch" on the Achilles during walking and thereby reduces the stress on the tendon.

The forces applied to the Achilles tendon during activities are proportional to body weight. Therefore losing weight (even a small amount) can be very helpful.

Surgical Treatment of Achilles Tendonitis

Surgical debridement, that is, the removal of the damaged tissue with meticulous repair of the remaining tendon, may be chosen if non-operative treatment fails. One setting where surgery may be considered more readily is that of a high-level athlete with insertional Achilles tendonitis and a Haglund's deformity. This surgery usually involves removing the prominent excess bone and the thickened inflamed retrocalcaneal bursa and debriding the Achilles tendon. In older, heavy-set middle-aged patients with insertional Achilles tendonitis that have truly failed a focused non-operative treatment regiment it may be necessary to transfer the Flexor Hallucis Longus (FHL) tendon into the calcaneus to help offload the Achilles.

Recovery from surgery can be prolonged. Initially, the leg is immobilized to allow the wound to heal. Once the wound is healed, gentle range of motion exercises can be started. Some patients are limited in weight-bearing for the first six weeks during the healing process. Gradually, activity can be increased. Improvement in strength continues for several months and may take over one year.

Stiffness of the ankle, rupture of the tendon, and deep vein thrombosis are known potential complications of surgery. Wound healing issues and infection can occur and when they do it is a very serious problem because loss of skin and soft-tissue in this area is very hard to treat.

RISK FACTORS AND PREVENTION

Regular calf stretching (Figures 6 & 7), can help improve the Achilles tendon's mechanical compliance ("stretchability" in layman's terms) and makes it more resilient.

Figure 6: Calf Stretching

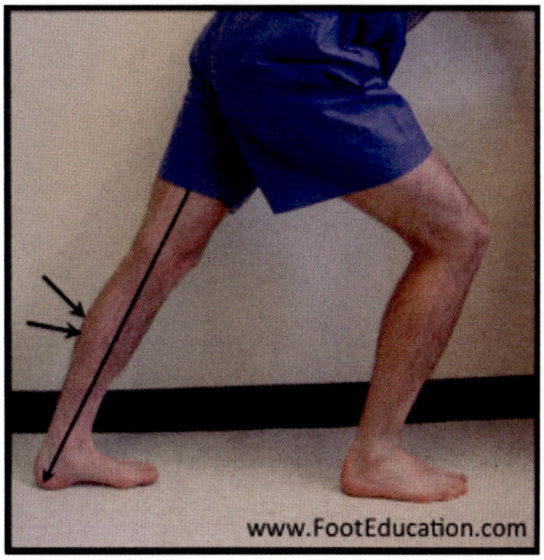

A consistent calf-stretching program is an important part of treatment and prevention of Achilles injuries (Figure 6). Leaning against the wall with one foot forward and the back heel kept on the ground will stretch the Achilles and posterior calf muscles. As it is the outer calf muscle (gastrocnemius) that is usually tight this stretch should be performed with the knee straight as the gastrocnemius originates from the posterior aspect of the distal femur. Bending the knee will take the tension off the gastrocnemius and place it on the soleus.

Figure 7: Eccentric Calf Stretching and Strengthening

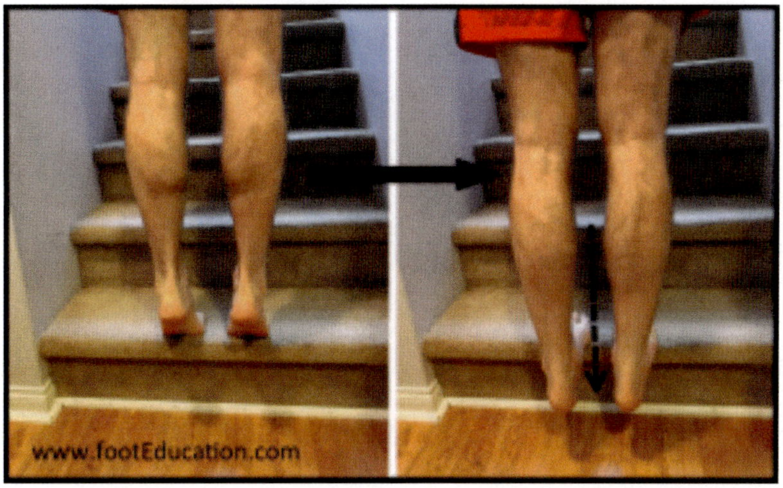

Controlled "eccentric" exercises where the Achilles tendon is being lengthened while the calf muscle contracts, may help prevent (or treat) Achilles tendonitis (Figure 7). This includes exercises such as the "Heel drop" shown here. In this exercise, patients stand on their toes while positioned on the edge of a ledge such as a stair. They then slowly lower their heels down below the ledge simultaneously stretching and strengthening the Achilles tendon. This can be done with both legs at a time (bilaterally) or for a more concentrated effort, one leg at a time. It can also be done with the knees straight (putting force on the gastrocnemius) or the knees bent (putting force on the soleus). Patients should gradually work up to performing 5 sets of 10 repetitions. These exercises should be performed 5-6 days per week during the active treatment phase and then 3 times per week to minimize the chance of developing recurrent symptoms. It is critical that this exercise is approached cautiously, as it has the potential to put excessive pressure on the Achilles. Patients should always warm up first (ex. get their blood flowing on an exercise bike for 5-10 minutes) before performing these exercises.

Using a heel lift or a shoe with a moderate heel can help reduce the stress on the tendon.

MISCELLANY

In Greek mythology Achilles was dipped into the River Styx by his mother Thetis to coat his body with a shield of protection. Thetis grasped Achilles by the heel (on the eponymous tendon) when she dipped him, leaving that one area not washed by the river, and in turn unprotected. From that comes the term "Achilles heel," connoting a person's area of vulnerability.

KEY TERMS

Achilles tendonitis, insertional Achilles tendonitis, non-insertional Achilles tendonitis, Haglund's deformity, retrocalcaneal bursitis

SKILLS

Bedside skills for the diagnosis of disorders of the Achilles include the ability to take a detailed but focused history and perform a thorough musculoskeletal examination.

CHAPTER 25.

ANKLE SPRAIN

DESCRIPTION

Ankle sprains are among the most common musculoskeletal injuries. Patients typically describe an episode where they "roll their ankle" to one side (often inward, a so called "inversion" sprain (Figure 1) and thereby tear the ligaments on the outside (lateral) ankle. This is contrasted with a less common "eversion" sprain where the foot rolls to the outside and the medial (deltoid) ligament is torn. Patients with sprained ankles can have significant pain and swelling. There is usually a limp, but unlike an ankle fracture, a sprained ankle will usually tolerate some weight-bearing but, in severe cases, not for 7 to 10 days. Although the phrase "it's just a sprain" may suggest that this is always a minor injury, ankle sprains can in rare cases lead to significant impairment. Expeditious treatment – directed at limiting swelling and regaining motion – helps ensure the best possible recovery.

Figure 1: Ankle Inversion, the typical mechanism of injury of an ankle sprain

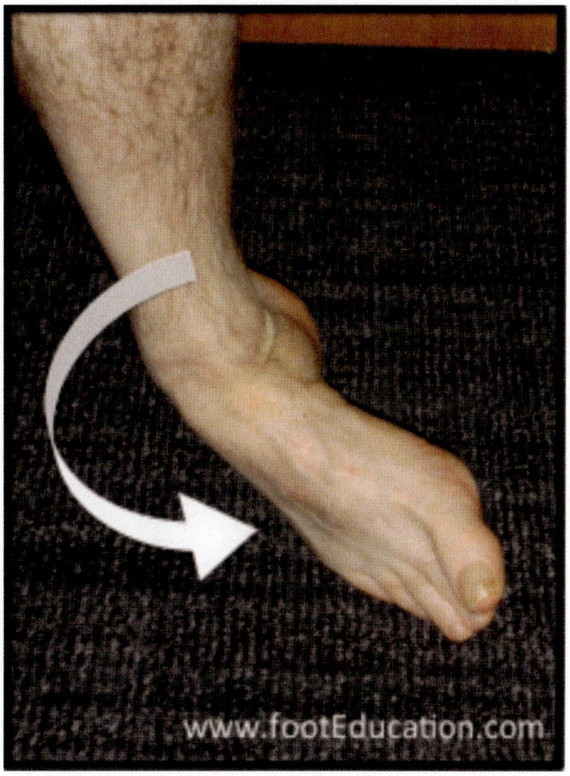

STRUCTURE AND FUNCTION

The ankle joint comprises the articulation of the tibia and fibula with the talus. However, the ligamentous constraints of the ankle also span the subtalar and talonavicular joints as well. The tibia and fibula are held together by the tibiofibular ligaments (anterior and posterior) and interosseous membrane, collectively known as the syndesmotic ligaments. These two bones form a mortise (inverted "U") into which the talus fits (Figure 2).

Figure 2: The Ankle Mortise. The talus (T) sits in an inverted U known as the mortise. The joint between the tibia (Tib) and fibula (Fib), the distal tibiofibular syndesosis. This relationship is vital to ankle function and is regulated by the anterior and posterior tibiofibular ligaments also referred to as the syndesmotic ligaments (shown in red). (Image courtesy of Joseph Bernstein MD)

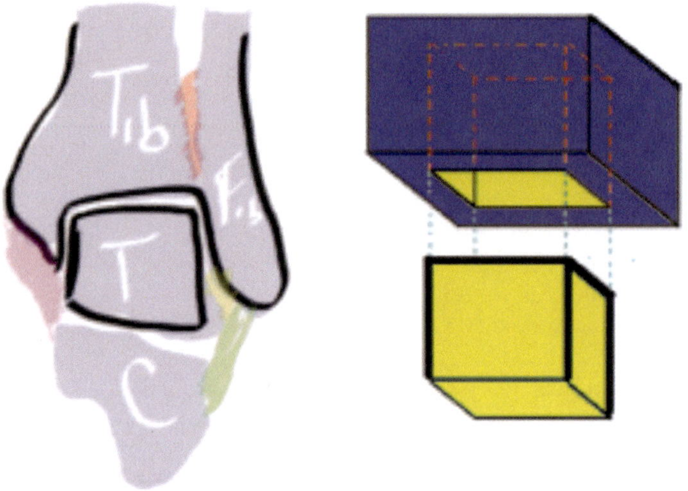

The talus, in turn, acts as a "universal joint" that is connected to the calcaneus, forming the subtalar joint.

In addition to the syndesmotic ligaments, the ankle joint is stabilized, on the lateral side by the anterior and posterior talo-fibular ligaments and the calcaneofibular ligament, together referred to as the *lateral collateral ligaments* (Figure 3).

Figure 3: The Lateral Ligaments of the Ankle.

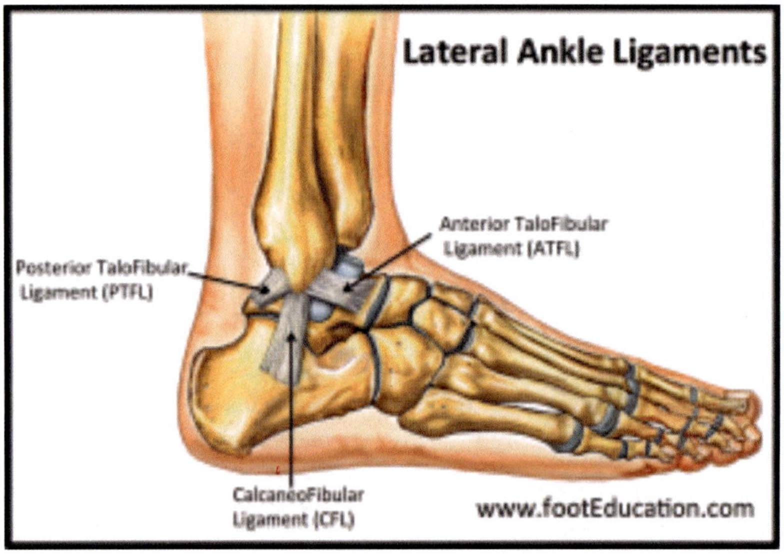

With its three parts, the deltoid ligament serves as the medial constraint of the ankle (Figure 4). The length and tension on these ligaments are vital to their role in the regulation of the *coupled motion* that occurs between the tibia, talus, calcaneus and navicular. The deeper branch of the ligament is securely fastened in the talus, while the more superficial, broader aspect runs into the calcaneus and navicular. Like the anterior talo-fibular ligament, the deltoid is rarely torn completely but rather becomes stretched (deformed) when stressed.

Figure 4: The Deltoid Ligament on the Medial Ankle The deltoid ligament is outlined in yellow (and shaped like a Delta). Within this ligament, there is a connection between the tibia and the navicular (blue), talus (red) and calcaneus (green). (Image courtesy of Joseph Bernstein MD)

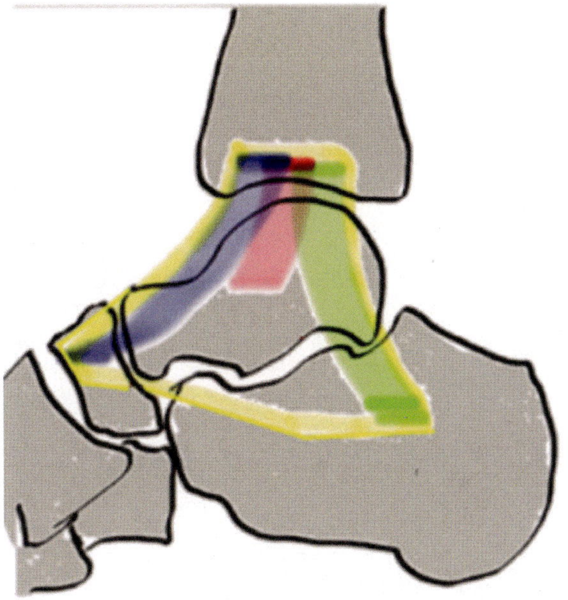

The anterior talo-fibular ligament (ATFL) is the ankle ligament most often sprained. The ATFL courses from the fibula to the neck of the talus and stabilizes the ankle joint against anterior translation. Inversion of the ankle is resisted by a combination of the ATFL and calcaneo-fibular ligament. The ATFL itself is not a distinct ligament but, rather a thickening of the lateral joint capsule. When it is sprained, the associated interstitial tearing may result in lengthening. This stretching may lead to symptomatic ankle instability.

The calcaneo-fibular ligament (CFL) originates at the tip of the fibula and courses distal and posterior inserting into the calcaneus. Unlike the ATFL, the CFL is a distinct ligamentous structure.

The posterior talo-fibular ligament (PTFL) originates from posterior margin of the fibula and inserts into the posterior talus. The PTFL stabilizes the ankle joint and the subtalar joint. Injuries to the PTFL are rare, unless there is an ankle dislocation or marked subluxation.

The anterior inferior tibio-fibular ligament is the one injured in a so-called "high ankle sprain." This ligament is positioned on the anterolateral aspect of the ankle and helps stabilize the mortise (Figure 5). Injuries to this ligament occur when the foot is stuck on the ground and rotates externally. A high ankle sprain can heal with irritating scar formation (hypertrophy–a condition known as anterior-lateral ankle impingement.

Figure 5: Anterior Inferior Tibiofibular Ligament

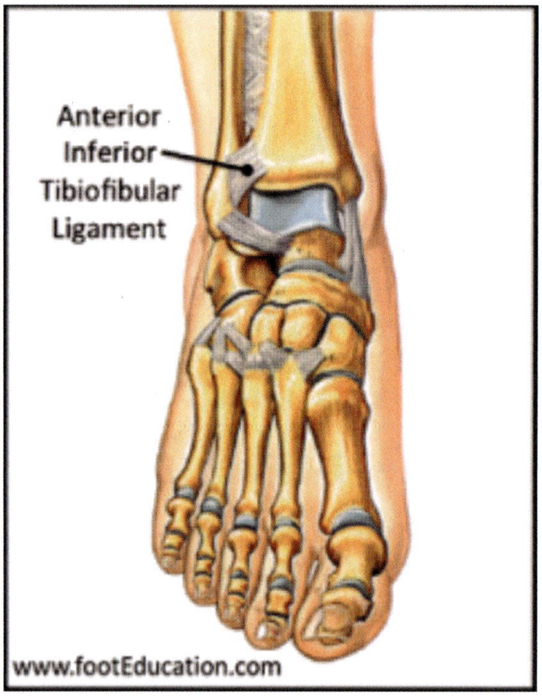

The interosseous membrane is composed of strong fibrous tissue that runs between and connects the tibia and fibula. The interosseous membrane along with the anterior or posterior syndesmotic ligaments can be torn in certain patterns of ankle fractures, in which the tibia and fibula spread apart, a so-called diastasis rendering the ankle unstable.

Collectively, the tibio-fibular ligament and the interosseous membrane are called the syndesmosis.

PATIENT PRESENTATION

Ankle Sprains

Patients with ankle sprains typically describe a twisting episode where they invert (or less often, evert) their ankle. Pain, swelling and difficulty ambulating are common.

A sprained ankle may often have associated redness due to the increased blood flow to this area (Figure 6). Without a history of an injury, this skin appearance may suggest cellulitis (infection of the skin). Physical examination of the acutely injured ankle will reveal swelling over the outer aspect of the ankle. There will be tenderness over the outer front (anterolateral) aspect of the ankle.

Figure 6: Ankle Swelling and Redness (erythema) Post-Ankle Sprain

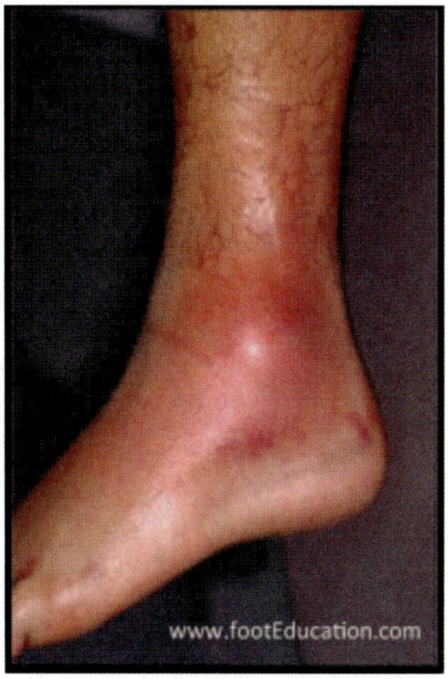

It is important to palpate the base of the anterior process of the calcaneus, the 5th metatarsal, the navicular and the Lisfranc joint for tenderness, as the same mechanism that creates an ankle sprain can lead to other injuries there as well.

As swelling and pain decreases, during the recovery period it may be possible to assess for ankle instability. Laxity of the ATFL is assessed with an anterior drawer maneuver (Figure 7). Integrity of the calcaneofibular ligament is assessed by inverting the foot while palpating the lateral talar dome. Either or both of these tests can be obscured by guarding due to pain. The anterior draw test is performed on both the injured and uninjured side to obtain comparison. The examiner assesses the amount of translation of the foot relative to the shin and also the "quality of the end point" (i.e., if a firm stop –a rope snapping to attention–is encountered).

Figures 7: The Ankle Drawer Test

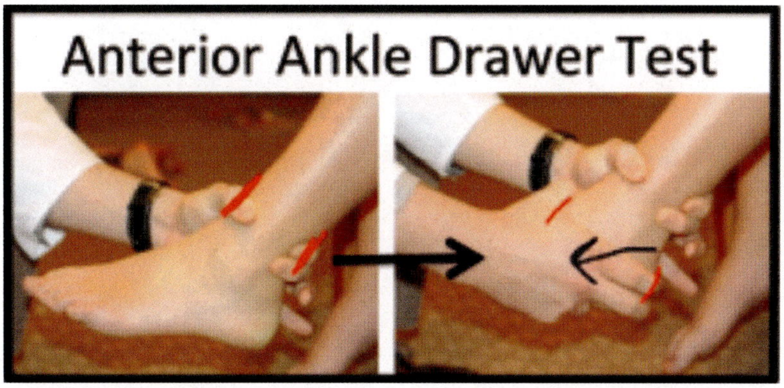

The anterior ankle drawer test is performed with the patient sitting on an exam table, with knees flexed and the foot dangling over the edge of the table. The examiner grasps and stabilizes the shin in one hand and applies anteromedial force to the heel with the other hand, using the deltoid ligament as a hinge.

High Ankle Sprains

So-called "high ankle sprains" are injuries to the syndesmosis, which lies between the tibia and fibula ("high") above the joint.

High ankle sprains are less common than lateral ankle sprains, but when they occur they are often more debilitating. They occur from a twisting injury to the ankle when the foot is planted on the ground. These injuries are produced by a sudden change of direction due to an externally applied force, as may be seen from a tackle in a football game. Pain located on the anterolateral aspect of the ankle is the main symptom. However, a high ankle sprain can also occur in combination with an inversion or eversion injury and therefore medial or lateral pain can be present as well.

The "squeeze test," namely compressing (squeezing) the tibia and fibula together approximately four inches above the ankle joint, can be used to detect a high ankle sprain. This test will tend to reproduce focal symptoms in patients who have had a high ankle sprain. The external rotation test, namely, holding the foot in dorsiflexion and then externally rotating it, will also reproduce focal symptoms when high ankle sprain is present.

OBJECTIVE EVIDENCE

X-rays should be obtained if there is bony tenderness on the posterior aspect of either malleoli or an inability to bear weight (Ottawa Ankle Rules). The x-rays should include the foot if there is tenderness on either the anterior process of the calcaneus, 5th metatarsal or the navicular. X-rays of the knee joint are needed if an isolated medial malleolus is detected on the initial film or if there is widening of the mortise (proximal fibular fracture can occur in combination with ankle injuries and must be ruled out).

X-rays must be examined to exclude not only fracture but diastasis, namely, an increased distance between the tibia and fibula implying damage to the syndesmosis.

Particular attention should be paid to ensure that the ankle joint mortise is symmetrical: the space between the talus and tibia medially should match the space laterally (Figure 8).

Figure 8: Talus Sits Squarely in the Mortise. The amount of space (arrows) should be uniform on all sides.

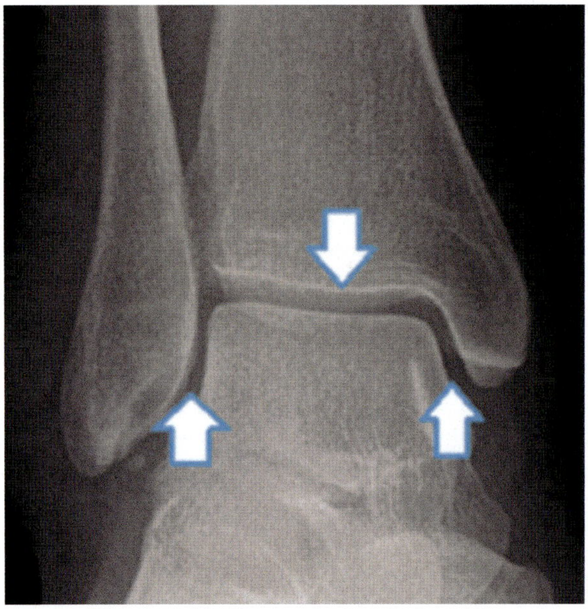

Stress x-rays – imaging the ankle while the heel is pushed towards one side while the leg is pushed in the opposite direction – may be used to assess instability in chronic cases. These films should be used only with great caution in the acute setting as the procedure may displace otherwise non-displaced injuries.

There is typically no role for MRI in acute ankle sprains. An MRI may be indicated in cases of chronic pain after a sprain. An MRI could detect a talar osteochondral injury or extra-articular sources of residual pain such as tendonitis or scarring of the restraining ligaments. Approximately 10% of severe ankle sprains may have associated injuries to the articular surface of the talus. An MRI may also be helpful in identifying an injury to the syndesmosis.

EPIDEMIOLOGY

According to Waterman et al (PMID: 20926721), emergency department data suggest an incidence rate of 2.15 ankle sprain per 1000 person/year in the United States, with a peak incidence rate more than triple that for teenagers between fifteen and nineteen years of age. The *overall* incidence rate by gender is about the same, though younger males and older females have higher rates than their female and male counterparts respectively. Nearly half of all ankle sprains seen were related to athletic activity.

DIFFERENTIAL DIAGNOSIS

The key element in the differential diagnosis of an acute ankle injury is discerning what was injured: which bones may have been broken and which ligaments may have been sprained. Note that combination injuries are not only possible but are common.

Bony tenderness on the anterior process of the calcaneus, base of the 5th metatarsal, or navicular suggests a fracture there.

Tenderness coursing up the lateral aspect of the leg may suggest a peroneal tendon injury.

The squeeze test and external rotation test may detect a high ankle sprain (anterior inferior tibia-fibular ligament injury).

Once the diagnosis of an ankle sprain is made, it can be further refined into a grade:

- *Grade 1 sprain:* the anterior talofibular ligament is injured but not elongated (and thus not prone to cause instability);
- *Grade 2 sprain:* the anterior talofibular ligament is partially torn resulting in stretching that may destabilize the joint; and
- *Grade 3 sprain:* a complete tear of the anterior talofibular ligament. Note that instability may be masked by swelling or guarding.

RED FLAGS

An inability to bear weight or tenderness in the bone (including the medial and lateral malleoli as well as the 5th metatarsal and navicular) signify a need for radiographs (as per the Ottawa Ankle Rules).

Blood on the skin suggests an open fracture.

TREATMENT OPTIONS AND OUTCOMES

The initial treatment of an ankle sprain is known by the mnemonic RICE. RICE is used to limit swelling, as too much swelling can significantly increase the patient's pain and ultimate recovery time.

- **R**est: minimize mobilization and activity in the initial recovery period.
- **I**ce: Apply ice, but not continuously. A regimen of 10 minutes on and 10 minutes off will minimize the risk of thermal injury to the skin.
- **C**ompression: This should be tight enough to decrease swelling but loose enough to allow the foot to be perfused.
- **E**levation: To be maximally effective, the foot should be held higher than the thigh, to allow gravity to

help drain the edema. Propping the foot in a stool or pillow is not apt to help drain fluid, but may help enforce rest and inactivity.

Non-Steroidal Anti-Inflammatory Drugs (NSAIDs) such as ibuprofen can be very helpful to decrease pain by decreasing the inflammatory response to the injury. However, there is some evidence that suggest that anti-inflammatories may have an adverse effect on ligament healing.

Once the symptoms associated with the initial ankle sprain have started to improve, patients will benefit from *physical therapy exercises* designed to improve their range of motion, strength and proprioception.

Proprioception is the ability of the brain to sense the position of a joint (ex. ankle) and control its movement relative to the rest of the body. Note that nerves within the ligament mediate proprioception and therefore this sense can be out of kilter following a ligament injury. As the acuity of the injury resolves, patients with seemingly normal ankles on examination (no swelling, no tenderness, no laxity) may still feel unstable if proprioception has not returned to normal. This is referred to as "functional instability."

"Figure of Eight" exercises are particularly helpful for regaining range of motion and proprioception. Patients should be instructed to imagine that the tip of their big toe is a pen and to then "draw" a figure of eight with the toe slowly, repeating the motion for 30-60 seconds. In the alternatives, patients can "sign" their names in script. It is important that the motion follow a deliberate pattern – and not random waving of the foot – as deliberate motion helps improve proprioception as well.

Proprioception can also be improved by having the patient stand on one foot with eyes closed. Once this is mastered, standing on one foot on a soft surface (such as a pillow or bed) with eyes closed and head moving side to side can further improve proprioception.

Rehabilitation after an ankle sprain can often be completed with a home program, though trained physical therapists may be beneficial in providing initial instruction defining the program.

Surgery is rarely indicated for the treatment of acute ankle sprains. However, patients who have recurrent ankle sprains may be candidates for an ankle ligament stabilization procedure to treat their anatomic instability and restore functional stability.

Most people with sprained ankles fully recover. Even if the ligaments are permanently deformed, the muscles crossing the ankle joint can provide sufficient dynamic stability. However, because ankle sprains are such a common injuries, even a low rate of complications (coupled with a high incidence) may produce a significant number of people with poor outcomes. Ankle injuries associated with chronic anatomic instability may lead to the development of traumatic arthritis.

RISK FACTORS AND PREVENTION

Risk factors for ankle sprains include a high arched foot (cavus foot), ligamentous laxity leading to increased inversion, participating in high risk activities (ex. basketball, soccer, volleyball), and a history of previous ankle sprains.

Rovere et al (PMID: 3132864) studied the effectiveness of taping, wearing a laced stabilizer and high-top or low-top shoes among collegiate football for 6 seasons. They reported that the combination associated with the fewest injuries overall was low-top shoes and laced ankle stabilizers.

MISCELLANY

Ankle sprains from playing basketball represent nearly 20% of all ankle sprains in the US. Football and soccer are the next most implicated sports causing ankle sprains during athletics.

KEY TERMS

Ankle sprain, syndesmosis, mortise, talo-fibular ligament, calcaneo-fibular ligament, deltoid ligament, proprioception

SKILLS

Recognize an ankle sprain and differentiate between it and other ankle and hindfoot injuries. Apply the Ottawa ankle rules to recognize need for x-rays.

CHAPTER 26.

CLAVICLE FRACTURES

DESCRIPTION

A clavicle fracture is a common injury seen after a fall on an outstretched arm or direct impact. A large majority of all clavicle fractures will occur in the middle third of the shaft. Traditionally, treatment was based on the premise that malunion (or even non-union) of clavicle fractures was well tolerated and imposed little morbidity. Accordingly, these fractures were usually treated with only a course of immobilization. Recently, that assumption has been questioned, and a greater number of clavicular fractures are currently treated operatively. Clavicular fractures that occur far laterally (known as distal clavicle fractures) must be considered distinctly, as they may involve the ligaments that suspend the glenohumeral joint. Also, because the clavicular physis is among the last to close (around age 21 or later), an apparent separation of the acromioclavicular joint in a young adult may actually represent a physeal fracture of the clavicle.

STRUCTURE AND FUNCTION

The clavicle (known colloquially as the collarbone), is a strut between the scapula (shoulder blade) and the sternum (breastbone).

Viewed from above, the clavicle is shaped like a capital "S", attaching medially to the sternum at the sternoclavicular joint, and laterally to the coracoid and the acromion. The inflexion point – the middle of the S – is the portion of the bone most prone to fracture.

The pectoralis major, sternocleidomastoid and deltoid muscles originate from the clavicle and the trapezius inserts on it (Figure 1).

Figure 1: The left clavicle as seen from above. The sternum is medial and the acromion is lateral. The points of muscular attachment are color-coded: medially, the sternocleidomastoid is red and the pectoralis is green; laterally the deltoid is yellow and the trapezius is orange. (modified from https://en.wikipedia.org/wiki/Clavicle#/media/File:Gray200.png)

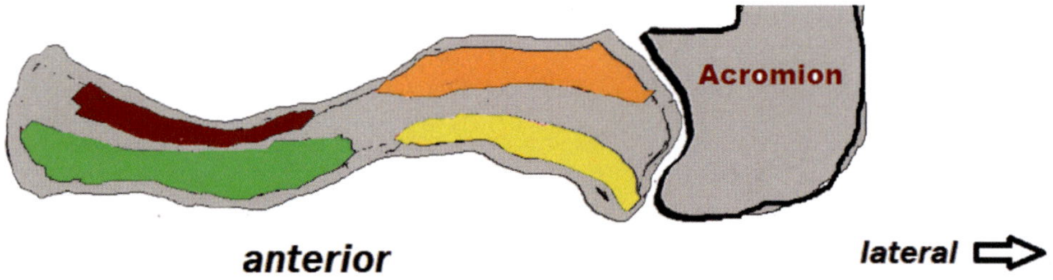

When the clavicle is fractured, the proximal (medial) portion can be pulled superiorly by the sternocleidomastoid muscles, while the distal portion is pulled inferiorly by the weight of the arm. The fracture fragments can also be displaced superiorly or posteriorly, leading to tenting and necrosis of the overlying skin or neurovascular injury, respectively.

The coracoclavicular ligaments, namely, the trapezoid and conoid, attach from the coracoid process to the inferior aspect of the clavicle and help suspend the arm. The acromioclavicular ligaments resist anterior/posterior displacement of the distal clavicle relative to the acromion. The clavicle overlies the brachial plexus, as well as the jugular and subclavian blood vessels.

PATIENT PRESENTATION

Clavicle fractures most commonly occur following a direct blow or after a fall on an outstretched arm. Patients will often report feeling a snapping sensation at the time of injury. Patients may present with the relative arm held by their other hand across the body in adduction. Movement of the arm will exacerbate the pain.

In the case of mid-shaft fractures, there may be a deformity of the fractured clavicle, with swelling and ecchymosis. Skin tenting from anterior displacement may be present as well. The proximal portion of the fractures may be pulled superiorly, while the distal portion may be pulled inferiorly.

Distal clavicle fractures (Figure 2) may present with no deformity, and tenderness around the acromioclavicular (AC) joint, similar to an AC joint separation.

Figure 2: A distal (lateral) clavicle fracture (red arrow) may be in the region (green star) of the ligaments that attached the clavicle to the scapula. (from https://radiopaedia.org/cases/22256)

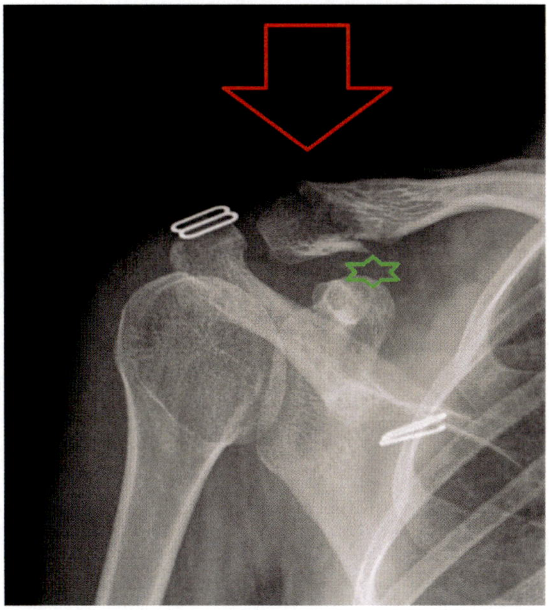

A neurovascular and respiratory exam is critical to rule out injury to the brachial plexus, subclavian vessels, or the lungs. Strength, sensation, pulses and difficulty of breathing should be assessed.

OBJECTIVE EVIDENCE

An anteroposterior chest radiograph showing both clavicles should be obtained if a clavicle fracture is expected. This can differentiate clavicle fractures from AC joint separations and sternoclavicular (SC) dislocations. The chest radiograph can also be used to assess for signs of vascular damage, such as a widened mediastinum and to rule out a pneumothorax.

Radiographs should also be obtained to rule out injuries to the glenohumeral joint and scapula. The required radiographs include the anterior-posterior (AP), axillary, and lateral ("scapular-Y") views. Most mid-shaft fractures can be visualized with this view.

Anteroposterior radiographs can best assess a clavicle fracture, especially in the proximal portion of the clavicle (Figure 3). A posteroanterior radiograph can be used to assess shortening of the clavicle for surgical planning (Figure 4). Computed tomography (CT) imaging can be utilized for evaluation of intra-articular involvement of the medial and lateral ends of the bone; CT is not needed for acute midshaft injuries.

Figure 3: A mid-shaft clavicle fracture (Case courtesy of A. Prof Frank Gaillard, https://radiopaedia.org/ From the case https://radiopaedia.org/cases/18050)

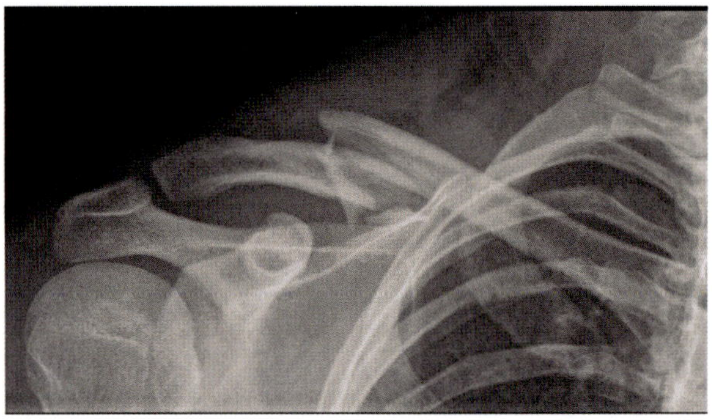

Figure 4: Figure 4: Shortening of the clavicle can be assessed by either of the following methods. On the left, the overlap between the ends of the medial and lateral fragments is measured directly; this is shown in red. At right, the entire medial-to-lateral length of both the injured and the normal clavicle are measured. As shown, the blue line represents the length of the shortened clavicle, the green line shows the length of the normal one, and the red line represents the difference. (from https://bmcmusculoskeletdisord.biomedcentral.com/articles/10.1186/s12891-017-1881-x)

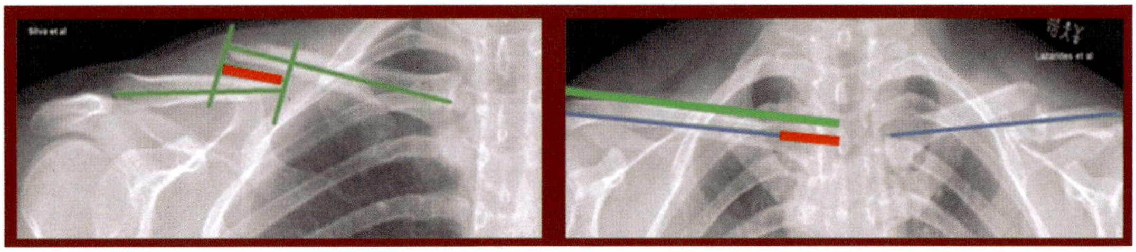

Arteriography may be helpful in evaluating vascular injury.

Clavicle fractures are classified by location. The regions of the clavicle are segmented into thirds: medial (aka proximal), middle and lateral (distal). Mid-shaft clavicular fractures represent an overwhelming majority of these injuries (80%). Among the distal clavicular fractures (close to the AC joint) the fractures are further classified (following the scheme of Neer) in terms of the location of the clavicle fracture relative to the coracoclavicular ligaments. These fractures are designated as medial to the coracoclavicular ligaments; between the two coracoclavicular ligaments (with an intact trapezoid ligament attached to the distal lateral segment); and lateral to coracoclavicular ligaments and thus extending into the acromioclavicular joint itself.

Clavicle fractures are also classified by the degree of displacement: nondisplaced; incompletely displaced (that is, some overlap of the fracture edges); and completely displaced.

EPIDEMIOLOGY

Clavicle fractures account for 2-5% of fractures in adults and 10-15% of fractures in the pediatric population. Approximately 70% of clavicle fractures occur in males. There is a bimodal distribution of age, with the highest rates of fracture in active patients below the age of 25 years old and patients above the age of 55 years old. Falls, motor vehicle accidents, and sports-related injuries are the most common causes of clavicle fractures in adults.

DIFFERENTIAL DIAGNOSIS

As with many traumatic injuries, the differential diagnosis narrows considerably after radiographs are obtained: the bone is either broken or it is not.

If there is no fracture, a clavicular contusion might be the diagnosis. The presentation is similar to that of a clavicle fracture with swelling, ecchymosis, tenderness and limited range of motion secondary to pain. Also, a ligament injury (especially in the form of an acromioclavicular joint separation) may be present. An acromioclavicular separation presents as pain over the acromioclavicular joint and distal shoulder. There may or may not be displacement of this joint. Sternoclavicular dislocation occurs after direct trauma to the chest wall and may present with deformity of the sternoclavicular joint and pain with arm movement. It is important to evaluate for fractures of the scapula, including the acromion and glenoid. If both the clavicle and glenoid neck are fractured, the glenohumeral joint has no connection to the axial skeleton. This is known as a "floating shoulder". These injuries are associated with neurovascular injury. Rib fractures can also occur concomitantly with clavicular fractures given the traumatic mechanism of injury.

RED FLAGS

Posterior or inferior displacement of a segment puts neurovascular structures, as well as the lungs, at risk of injury.

Paresthesia, sensory deficits, strength deficits and/or abnormal reflexes in the relative arm may indicate an injury to the brachial plexus or one of its nerve branches.

Pulselessness, asymmetric pulses or coldness of limb may indicate an injury of the subclavian artery or vein.

Difficulty breathing and chest pain may indicate the presence of rib fractures, a hemothorax (vascular trauma), or a pneumothorax.

TREATMENT OPTIONS AND OUTCOMES

Immobilization is indicated for fractures that are no more than minimally displaced – the majority of clavicle fractures. With this injury, the patient is initially placed in a sling, with gentle range of motion exercises started at ~2 weeks post injury, when patients are able to move the arm without pain. Strengthening exercises can be started 6 to 10 weeks after injury, when there is radiographic evidence of healing. Return to contact sports is typically allowed after 4 to 5 months, when there is radiographic evidence of fracture union.

Patients with clavicle fractures that are completely displaced and foreshortened by 2 cm or more are commonly indicated for surgery (Figure 5). If the ends of the fracture are not in contact and the clavicle is shortened by 2 cm or more, the risk of non-union increases. This rationale is controversial, in the sense that delayed open treatment can be reserved for symptomatic non-unions and malunions. Also, not every patient with a displaced and foreshortened fracture will be sufficiently symptomatic to warrant further treatment.

Figure 5: A clavicle fracture fixed with a plate. (from https://bmcmusculoskeletdisord.biomedcentral.com/articles/10.1186/1471-2474-15-380)

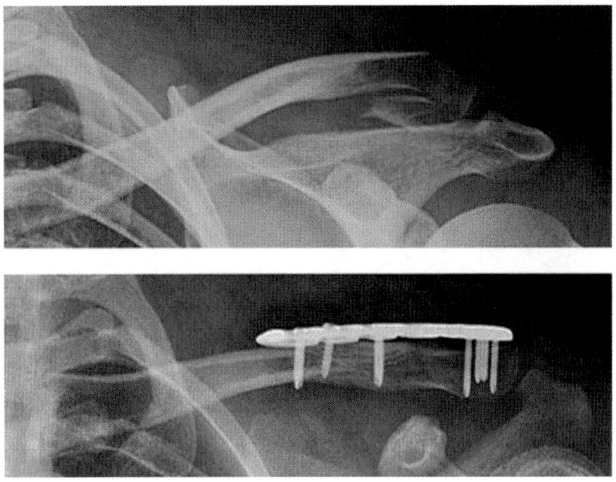

Any displacement of distal third fractures may be an indication for surgical treatment as the displacement implies a concomitant ligament injury and higher risk of non-union.

Urgent open treatment is indicated for open fracture (or skin tenting), with subclavian artery or vein injury, or when there is a scapular fracture as well (the so-called floating shoulder).

Polytrauma may also be an indication for open treatment for a fracture that, in isolation, would be indicated for closed treatment.

Open reduction and internal fixation can utilize intramedullary rods, or plates and screws. After internal fixation, patients are immobilized in a sling for 2 weeks; during this time passive range of motion exercises are performed. Rehabilitation is similar to non-op management.

While patient satisfaction and shoulder function is typically high following non-operative immobilization, there is a risk of malunion and nonunion. The risk of nonunion increases with increasing amounts of displacement.

Non-operative treatment is also associated with higher rates of cosmetic dissatisfaction compared to operative treatment.

Open reduction and internal fixation is associated with shorter time to union and better functional recovery. Compared to closed reduction and immobilization, surgical fixation results in significantly better outcomes 6 weeks after injury, but this difference dissipates after about 6 months. Unfortunately, there is a high complication rate, as high as 34%, and a significant reoperation rate, ranging from 18-25%. (Often, the second surgery is for hardware removal, not failure of the first operation.)

RISK FACTORS AND PREVENTION

Athletic involvement increases the risk for clavicle fracture. The use of protective equipment when participating in contact sports may decrease the risk of clavicle fracture.

MISCELLANY

For about 2,390 out of the last 2400 years, non-operative treatment of clavicular fractures was the norm. In 400 BC, Hippocrates wrote this about clavicle fractures: “Patients attach much importance to it, as supposing the mischief greater than it really is, and the physicians bestow great pains in order that it may be properly bandaged; but in a little time the patients, having no pain, nor finding any impediment to their walking or eating, become negligent; and the physicians finding they cannot make the parts look well, take themselves off, and are not sorry at the neglect of the patient, and in the meantime the callus is quickly formed." Likewise, in 1994, Mullaji and Jupiter (Injury. 25(1):41-5, 1994 Jan) said this: "Internal fixation of the clavicle is rarely necessary."

It was not until 2007 that the Canadian Orthopedic Trauma Society wrote: "Operative fixation of a displaced fracture of the clavicular shaft results in improved functional outcome and a lower rate of malunion and nonunion compared with nonoperative treatment." (Journal of Bone & Joint Surgery – American Volume. 89(1):1-10, 2007)

Clavicle fractures are the most common fractures in newborns. Many of these injuries are diagnosed after the baby and mother are discharged from the hospital post-partum. Brachial plexus injuries can also occur during these fractures, but almost always resolve.

KEY TERMS

Clavicle, collar bone, fracture, open reduction, immobilization

SKILLS

Perform an upper extremity musculoskeletal exam with concern for neurovascular injury. Interpret radiographs of the chest and shoulder for clavicle fractures, as well as other concerning signs such as rib fractures or widened mediastinum. Apply a sling or figure-of-eight brace to a patient.

CHAPTER 27.

PROXIMAL HUMERUS FRACTURES

DESCRIPTION

The proximal humerus comprises four "parts": the greater tuberosity, the lesser tuberosity, the humeral head and the humeral shaft. Fractures in this area are common, especially among older patients. Among elderly patients with osteoporotic bone, low-energy falls are the most common mechanism of injury; younger individuals sustain fractures of the proximal humerus from high-energy trauma, and may have concomitant injuries. Many proximal humerus fractures are amenable to nonoperative treatment. On the other hand, because displacement can upset the mechanics of the glenohumeral joint (with or without concomitant tearing of the rotator cuff) or disrupt the blood supply to the head, surgery may be needed in that setting. Management of displaced proximal humerus fractures remains controversial. Surgical indications are based on multiple factors including patient age, handedness, functional demands and evidence of pre-existing glenohumeral arthritis or rotator cuff pathology.

STRUCTURE AND FUNCTION

As shown in Figure 1 and 2, there are four bony "parts" of the proximal humerus. These represent the coalescence of distinct ossification centers and thus are prone to separation during injury. There are two regions designated as a "neck" of the proximal humerus. The "anatomical neck", representing the fused epiphyseal plate, is above the tuberosities and below the articular surface. The "surgical neck" is the junction between the shaft and the tuberosities. The region between the greater and lesser tuberosities is not a "neck"; rather, it is denoted as the "bicipital groove." This groove is so named because it houses the long head of the biceps as it begins its course down the arm.

Figure 1: The four osseous segments are humeral head and articular surface (1), greater tuberosity (2), lesser tuberosity (3) and humeral shaft (4). The so-called anatomic neck is shown in green; this represents the fused epiphyseal plate below the articular surface. The so-called surgical neck is shown in blue. This is the junction between the shaft and the tuberosities. The bicipital groove lies between the greater and lesser tuberosities.

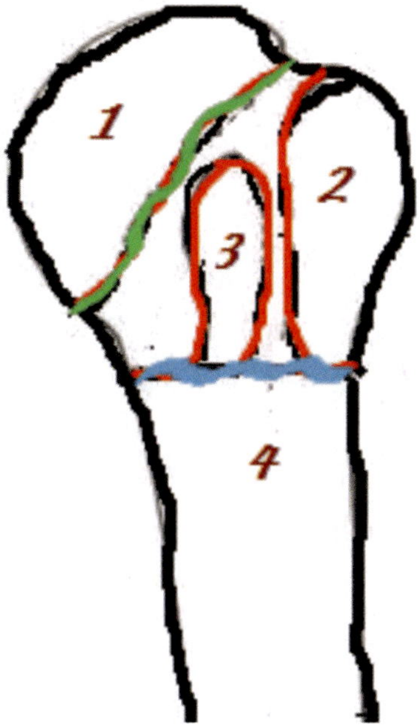

Figure 2: An x-ray highlighting the articular surface (blue), greater tuberosity (red), lesser tuberosity (yellow) and humeral shaft (green).

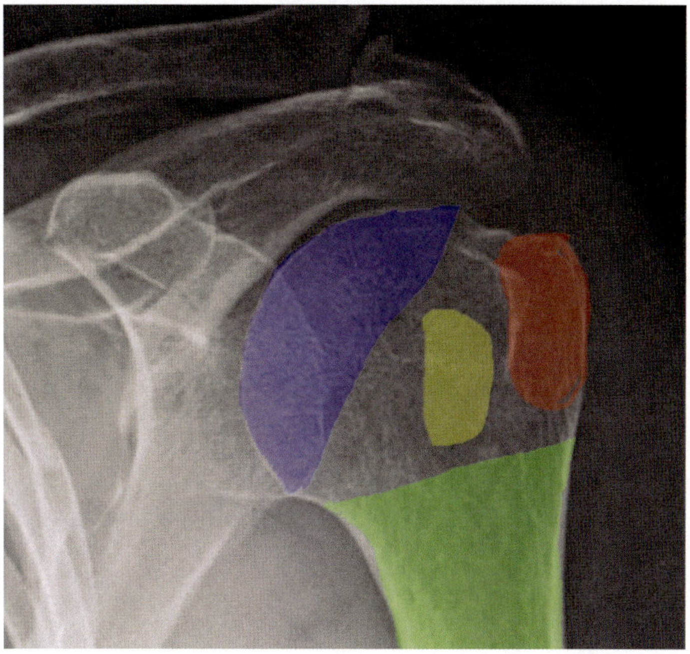

There are multiple muscular insertions on the proximal humerus. These attachments typically work in tandem to produce balanced forces that stabilize the glenohumeral joint. With a fracture, though, they can be deforming.

Important insertions include: The supraspinatus, infraspinatus, and teres minor insertion on the greater tuberosity. These assist with abduction and external rotation and with fracture, can cause superior and posterior displacement of the greater tuberosity.

The subscapularis inserts on the lesser tuberosity and exerts an internal rotation force. With fracture, the subscapularis displaces the lesser tuberosity medially.

Pectoralis major inserts on the lateral margin of the bicipital groove, distal and lateral to the lesser tuberosity and can displace the shaft medially and anteriorly.

The deltoid inserts on the shaft distal to the greater tuberosity and abducts the humeral shaft.

The major blood supply to the proximal humerus is from the anterior and posterior humeral circumflex arteries. Fractures of the anatomical neck can lead to osteonecrosis if the vascular supply of the humeral head is disrupted.

The axillary nerve comes off the posterior cord of the brachial plexus. It then courses in an anterior and inferior direction lying just medial to the joint on the anterior aspect of the subscapularis. It then courses posteriorly, inferior to the glenohumeral joint. This nerve is susceptible to injury by traction when the humeral head comes out of place (either by fracture, dislocation or subluxation), owing to its relatively fixed position close to the inferior capsule.

PATIENT PRESENTATION

Patients present with a known history of trauma.

The mechanism of injury typically varies based on age. For elderly patients, the history usually involves a low energy fall from a standing height. Younger patients often present following a high-energy trauma with a direct blow to the shoulder. Less commonly, proximal humerus fractures may occur as the result of a violent muscle contraction (i.e. during a seizure or following an electrical shock).

Initial complaints include pain and immobility of the affected upper extremity. Patients may report paresthesias or diminished sensation distal to the injury.

Complaints of weakness may be secondary to pain inhibition or possible nerve injury.

Patients will often present with the affected upper extremity held closely to the chest by the contralateral hand (to minimize painful motion).

Swelling of the affected limb appears within hours after injury. Bruising along the arm and chest wall (ecchymoses) might not appear until a few days after injury.

With a fracture, inspection may reveal subtle derangement of the normal contours of the shoulder, but gross deformity is rare.

Important elements of the history include the mechanism of injury. In the case of a fall, for instance, a syncopal event or history suggestive of a seizure would warrant further workup.

A careful neurovascular exam should be conducted with particular attention to the axillary nerve. This may be assessed by presence of sensation on the lateral aspect of the proximal arm overlying the deltoid. Motor testing (i.e. assessing deltoid and teres minor function) is often not possible at initial presentation due to pain.

OBJECTIVE EVIDENCE

Three radiographs, a true A-P of the proximal humerus, a lateral (also known as a "scapular-Y" view) and an axillary view, should be obtained.

The A-P and lateral views are best for evaluation of the humerus. The axillary view is used to exclude dislocation/subluxation of the glenohumeral articulation.

If an axillary view cannot be obtained due to pain, Velpeau axillary view can be obtained which is done with the patient in a sling, leaning obliquely backward 45 degrees over the cassette. The beam is then directed caudally, orthogonal to the cassette.

Radiographs are used to classify the fracture in terms of the displacement of the parts affected. According to the system popularized by Neer (based on the original work by Codman), a broken part is designated provided it is displaced by 1 cm or more, or if there is 45 degrees or more of angulation.

(This classification has been criticized because it is not very reliable–two readers will often disagree on how many parts there are. On the other hand, the classification is powerful in that it reflects important clinical differences in terms of prognosis and treatment requirements, and thus it is still widely used. Because of the difficulty with x-ray interpretation, the text here will use line drawings and not clinical x-rays.)

"One-part fractures" (which seems to be a contradiction in terms) have no displaced fragments. A fracture without displaced fragments is a "one-part", regardless of the number of fracture lines.

"Two-part fractures" (Figure 3) have one displaced fragment. Typically, the displaced fragment is either the greater tuberosity or the shaft (with a fracture across the surgical neck). Rarely, the isolated fragment is the lesser tuberosity. This latter pattern is associated with posterior dislocation.

Figure 3: Various "two-part" fractures.

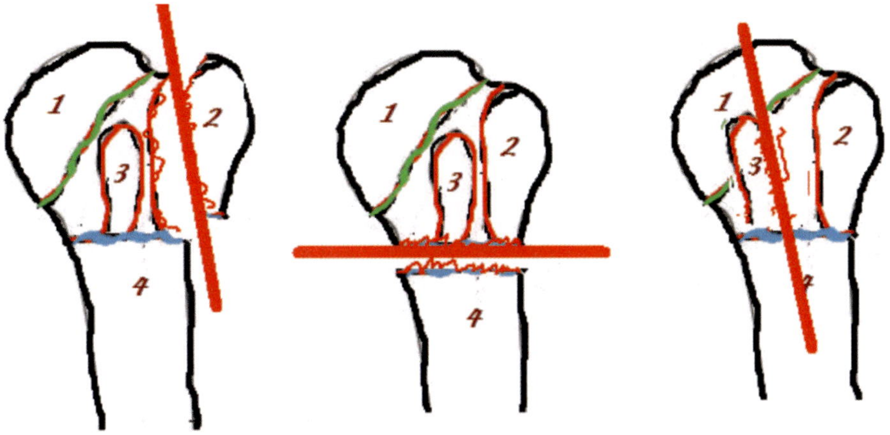

Figure 4: A "three-part" fracture.

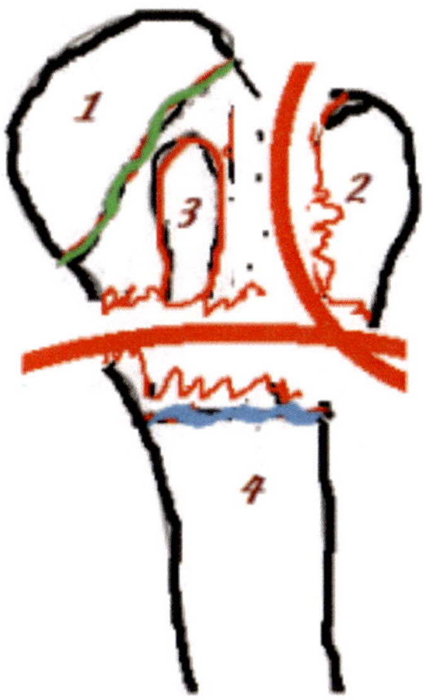

"Four-part fractures" (Figure 5) have displacement across fracture lines between all four parts

Figure 5: A "four-part" fracture.

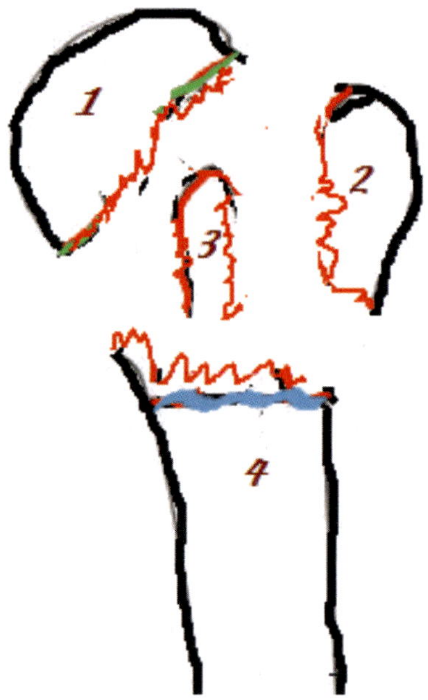

In addition, injuries can include fractures of the articular surface (head-splitting fractures and impaction fractures) and disruption of the glenohumeral articulation (fracture dislocation).

CT-scan may be helpful in evaluating articular involvement, degree of displacement, impression fractures and glenoid rim fractures. It can also be helpful when obtaining an axillary view is not possible.

MRI is usually not indicated unless rotator cuff integrity needs to be assessed.

Caveat: The Neer/Codman classification is used ubiquitously, though it was seen to have fairly low reliability (~50%) in reported studies. Unfortunately, CT scans do not help much either. That might be a function of the arbitrary criteria of 1 cm and 45 degrees. It may be best to "overcall" displacement in some cases: for example, treating a one-part greater tuberosity fracture as a two-part fracture, as the fragment can easily impinge even if only 9mm or 40 degrees displaced.

EPIDEMIOLOGY

Proximal humerus fractures comprise about 5% of all fractures. The incidence is 300,000 per year. Mechanism is either through a high energy trauma in younger individuals or low-energy falls in the elderly. Older individuals will sustain a fracture from a fall especially if there is underlying osteoporosis. More than 2/3 of proximal humeral fractures are sustained by females. Most proximal humerus fractures (85%) are nondisplaced.

DIFFERENTIAL DIAGNOSIS

The list of possible diagnoses that could explain the typical presentation of a proximal humerus fracture include a shoulder dislocation, an AC joint separation or a scapular, spinal or rib injury. Note that especially in high-energy trauma patients, concomitant injuries are common. Thus, the presence of a proximal humerus fracture does not exclude a second musculoskeletal diagnosis. It is also important to exclude the diagnosis of pneumothorax and hemothorax; axillary, suprascapular, or brachial plexus nerve injury; and axillary artery damage. Damage to the rotator cuff is common with displaced fractures.

RED FLAGS

Proximal humerus fractures with open wounds (or impending open-wounds, e.g. tenting of the skin by bone fragments) require urgent orthopaedic intervention.

Patients may report paresthesias or diminished sensation due to diffuse swelling; a detailed neurovascular assessment is warranted especially in the setting of such symptoms. The most commonly injured nerve is the axillary nerve and it can be tested even without moving the shoulder by assessing sensation over the deltoid muscle and verifying at least isometric deltoid contraction.

Peripheral pulses may remain palpable due to collateral circulation. A vascular injury may be suspected due to mechanism or signs of expanding hematoma.

A fracture from a simple fall from a standing height suggests osteoporosis, as well as underlying diseases that cause falling.

A visible indentation of the skin under the acromion (a subacromial sulcus) may suggest dislocation of the glenohumeral joint.

TREATMENT OPTIONS AND OUTCOMES

Minimally displaced fractures (one-part fracture) can be treated with a short course of immobilization in a sling (10-14 days) with early shoulder motion in the form of pendulum exercises thereafter. Passive motion or active-assisted range of motion therapy is best deferred until bony union has occurred (typically 6 to 12 weeks post-injury).

The treatment of two-part fractures depends on which parts are involved. Anatomic neck fractures, often associated with disruption of the blood supply, are difficult to treat without surgery. By contrast, surgical neck and lesser tuberosity fractures can usually heal adequately with non-operative treatment. Greater tuberosity two-part fractures are more likely to need surgical fixation, either to repair the rotator cuff dysfunction that accompanies the fracture or to prevent impingement of a fragment with superior translation.

Management of three-part and four-part proximal humerus fractures is dependent on multiple factors and precise surgical indications are not yet defined. Most displaced three-part and four-part fractures in physiologically younger patients are managed with surgery. Non-operative management of patients with lower functional demands can be successful as well.

Surgical treatment options include the following:

With closed reduction and percutaneous fixation, the fracture is reduced under fluoroscopic guidance and wires are inserted percutaneously. The aim is to stabilize the fracture enough to allow motion without excessive surgical dissection. The axillary nerve, cephalic vein and posterior humeral circumflex artery are all at risk with this technique. Also, closed reduction and percutaneous fixation is not apt to work in osteoporotic bone or if there is comminution. Lastly, a second operation may be necessary for pin removal.

Open reduction and internal fixation may also be used (Figure 6). Here, after the proximal humerus fracture is exposed, the fragments are reduced. This is then followed by internal fixation with either plates or sutures.

Figure 6: Proximal humerus fracture before (left) and after (right) surgical fixation. (courtesy of Jaimo Ahn, MD, PhD, FACS)

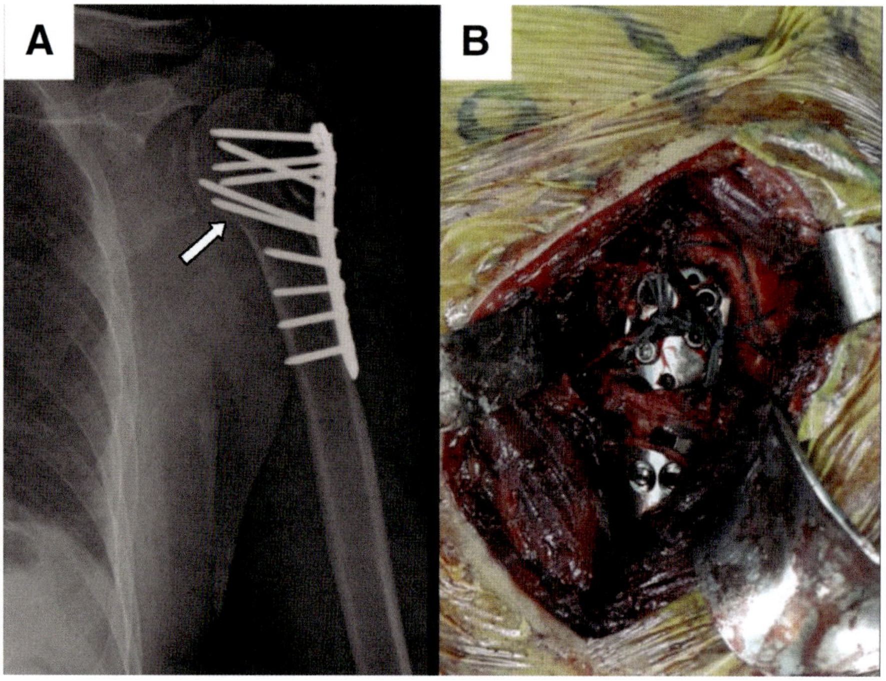

Locking plates are commonly used in the proximal humerus. Plate fixation is often augmented by sutures.

The use of an intramedullary device is a less invasive approach, as a full dissection is not needed; but of course it must be recalled that inserting the nail requires violation of the supraspinatus insertion (or if a more medial starting point is chosen, the superior articular surface itself).

Fractures that are unlikely to heal well (especially when the humeral head is not salvageable or there is extensive pre-existing arthritis) can be addressed with conventional joint replacement or reverse total shoulder replacement (Figures 7 and Figure 8). The latter is chosen when there is deficiency of the rotator cuff.

Figure 7: A proximal humerus fracture treated with hemiarthroplasty. (courtesy Andrew F. Kuntz, MD)

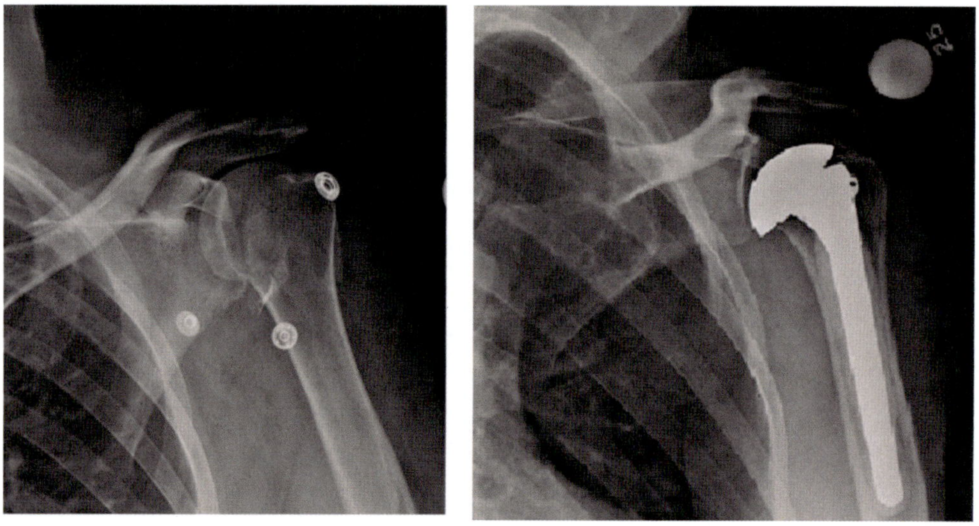

Figure 8: A proximal humerus fracture treated with a reverse hemiathroplasty. (courtesy Andrew F. Kuntz, MD)

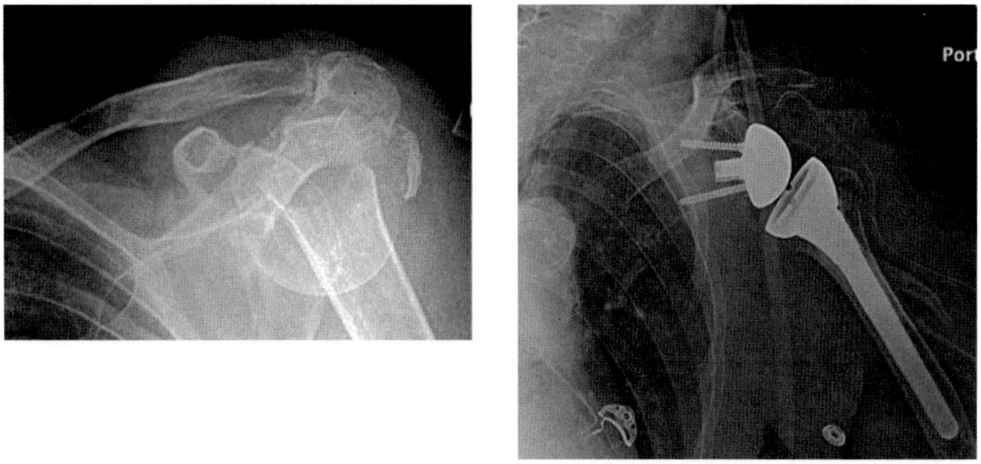

Although non-operative management might result in some degree of malunion or lost motion, a non-operative approach may still be desirable in some low-demand patients. Non-operative management of course avoids the costs and potential complications associated with operative intervention, and some loss of motion or deformity is usually well-tolerated by low-demand patients.

In general, nondisplaced proximal humerus fractures heal reliably with good functional return.

Displaced fractures that require surgery have less favorable outcomes. Even with full healing, there is often some component of arthrofibrosis and lost motion.

Four-part fractures are at especially high risk of developing osteonecrosis due to disruption of the blood supply to the head.

Proximal humerus fractures can have a significant detrimental effect on patient's quality of life beyond the issue of arm function. Shoulder injuries have a tendency to disrupt sleep, for example, and it may be difficult to shower during the period of healing.

Poor bone quality in the form of osteopenia or osteoporosis is a major risk factor for proximal humerus fracture. Accordingly, some patients with this fracture survive the shoulder injury but then go on to have another, more devastating fracture elsewhere (e.g., the hip).

RISK FACTORS AND PREVENTION

Osteoporosis and falling are the prime (modifiable) risk factors for proximal humerus fracture. Risk reduction involves maintenance of adequate bone mineral density (BMD) and decreasing the risk of falls. In osteopenic or osteoporotic patients, pharmacological therapy including calcium and vitamin D supplementation as well as bisphosphonates and other drug treatments have been shown to be effective in reducing the risk of fractures. For patients with comorbidities who place them at risk of falling (such as stroke), occupational therapy can be useful.

MISCELLANY

The classification of proximal humeral fractures is often associated with Dr. Charles Neer, but Dr. Neer himself credited E. A. Codman (Figure 9). Codman had many accomplishments (including the notion of collecting open data, the accomplishment that The CODMAN Group [publisher of this text] honors) but his anatomic analysis of the proximal humerus is among the larger ones.

Figure 9: Ernest Amory Codman, M.D. (Wikipedia)

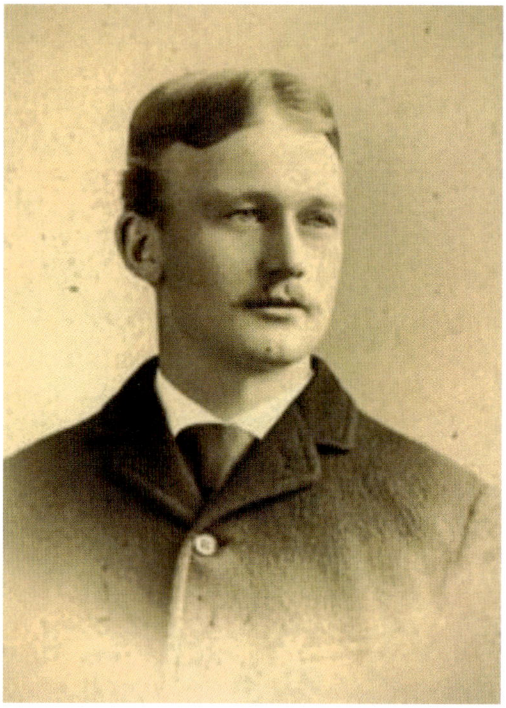

KEY TERMS

Greater tuberosity, lesser tuberosity, surgical neck, anatomic neck, axillary nerve, osteonecrosis, closed reduction, total shoulder arthroplasty

SKILLS

Describe fracture patterns as seen on plain x-rays. Perform a neurologic examination of the upper extremity, assessing the relevant sensory dermatomes, and motor testing of the muscle groups associated with the radial, median, ulnar, anterior interosseus, posterior interosseous, musculocutaneous and axillary nerves.

Made in the USA
Las Vegas, NV
23 November 2025

34989401R00124